Aeromedicine for Aviators

Aeromedicine for Aviators

KEITH E. E. READ

V.R.D., M.A., M.B., B.CHIR., M.R.C.O.G.

Surgeon Lieutenant Commander, Royal Naval Reserve
Authorized Medical Examiner, U.K. Civil Aviation
Member, British Medical Pilots Association
Member, Aerospace Medical Association, Washington, D.C.

FOREWORD BY

REX A. SMITH

Former Chairman, British Light Aviation Centre

Airlife

England

Read, Keith E. E.
    Aeromedicine for aviators.
    1. Aviation medicine
    I. Title
    616.9'80213   RC1062

    ISBN 1-85310-021-8

Published 1988 by Airlife Publishing Ltd.

First Airlife edition published 1976.

First published 1971
by Pitman Publishing.

Printed in England by Livesey Ltd., Shrewsbury.

Airlife Publishing Ltd.

7 St. John's Hill, Shrewsbury, England.

To
Flight Safety

I keep six honest serving-men
(They taught me all I knew);
Their names are What and Why and When
And How and Where and Who.
  The Elephant's Child, RUDYARD KIPLING

There are old pilots and there are bold
pilots, but there are no old, bold pilots.

ANON

Foreword

The British Light Aviation Centre has for a long time been concerned at the lack of any reliable, expert information on the aeromedical aspects of General Aviation. It is only in recent years that this important subject has begun to be appreciated by the private pilot.

The availability, therefore, of a book written in simple terms by a doctor who is also an active private pilot is particularly welcome. We commend Dr Read's book to all private pilots and hope that it will lead to a better understanding of this important, and often neglected, aspect of Flight Safety in private and light aviation.

We welcome it with enthusiasm and recommend all those that fly light aircraft to spend some time learning a little more of aeromedicine for their own good and indeed for the good of those with whom they may fly.

R. A. SMITH

Chairman
British Light Aviation Centre

Preface

Although this book has been written primarily for private pilots and glider pilots in the interests of flight safety, it is hoped that it will also be of use to professional pilots and airline crews. The physiological aspects of flight are explained, where possible in layman's language. No attempt has been made to go into the details of such a vast subject, but the book is offered as an addition to the knowledge a pilot requires to allow him to fly safely at all times.

K. E. E. READ
1970

Acknowledgments

The author wishes to acknowledge the generous help and encouragement he has received from Dr Geoffrey Bennett, The Chief Medical Officer, Civil Aviation Medical Department, The Board of Trade, London, W.C.2. This book could not have been written without the aid of my good friend, Steve Warwick-Fleming, himself a powered pilot and Gold "C" Glider pilot. Finally but by no means least, the author wishes to express his gratitude to his secretary, Miss Eileen Smith, for her patience and kindness in supplying innumerable cups of coffee and tea well into the silent hours when most of this book was written.

The quotation from *The Elephant's Child* is reproduced by permission of Mrs George Bambridge and Messrs Macmillan & Co, Ltd, London. Tables 3, 4 and 5 presented on pages 18, 19 and 20 are reproduced from Documenta Geigy Scientific Tables, 6th Edition, by permission of J. R. Geigy S.A., Basle, Switzerland.

Contents

1. Birds, Pilots and Doctors

Birds fly by instinct, whilst man flies by intelligence. Birds possess powers of navigation unknown to man and some flying mammals, like the bat, have a radar capability. Surface sensors provide birds with an exact knowledge of the state of air flow over their wings, and by using command centres in their brains they can alter the position of their feathers to act as flaps and lower their legs and feet to act as airbrakes. Their power/weight ration enables them to fly in a manner which will always be denied to man. The **Vestibular Apparatus** of a bird is adapted to flight and allows correct response to acceleration forces experienced whilst on the wing; even the ear drum of a bird is constructed to act like a variometer or vertical speed indicator. Man has learned to fly only in the past 200 years—at first in balloons and more recently, in heavier-than-air machines. Thus, a bird is a well-integrated aviator, wholly complete in itself and fed with exact knowledge of its air speed, angle of attack and attitude in yaw, pitch and roll from many sensors, of which vision is only one. In order to fly, man has had to surround himself with an aerofoil and since all his sensors, except vision, are unreliable in the air he has had to invent instruments to tell him visually what birds know instinctively from their multiple peripheral sensors.

Whilst a bird starts to fly when only a few weeks old, man must wait until he has grown up before he can learn to acquire this alien art. Thus for man to fly, intelligence and aptitude are required—and for man to fly safely, emotional stability must be wedded to mental capacity. It is only reasonable, under these circumstances, to require that an individual should attain

1

certain defined standards of mental and physical fitness before being allowed to learn to fly and that a pilot should be examined at regular intervals to ensure that his fitness standards have not deteriorated. An **Aviation Medical Examination** will include a review of the candidate's previous medical history, exact details of his immediate medical state and a thorough physical examination to assess his present medical fitness. The medical examiner's concern will be to satisfy himself that the candidate's **Central Nervous System**, which will include eyesight, reaches a satisfactory standard of performance. It is of vital importance to know whether the candidate has ever suddenly lost consciousness, or indeed whether he has ever had an **Epileptic Fit** or whether there is any family history of epileptiform seizures. Such an occurrence, whilst flying, could prove disastrous and involve the loss of many lives. Fortunately, it is possible to assess a predisposition to epilepsy by recording brain wave patterns. This is done by the **Electro-Encephalogram** (EEG). It is possible, with this apparatus, to diagnose brain damage due to various causes which will include traumatic injury, hypoxia, tumours and epilepsy, which may be either latent or overt. It is not unknown for individuals who have never had an attack of epilepsy before but who can be shown to have a tendency to epilepsy on the EEG to suffer a fit for the first time in the air and for this fit to be triggered off by **"Photic Phenomena"** produced by an aeroplane's propeller or by the rotor blades of a helicopter. Flickering lights of similar frequency may be produced by projectors of a type used in the early days of the cinema or by ski-ing down a tree-lined forest clearing. In the Royal Air Force all intending aircrew have an EEG before starting initial flying training. This examination will allow the Medical Department to prevent potential epileptics from ever flying and will also provide a base line for future reference should another examination be necessary at a later date, either because of head injury or brain damage or from any other cause such as deterioration of flying skill. For the Student Pilot or Private Pilot in civilian life an EEG is not, as yet, required unless the medical examiner feels this should be done for reasons which will include the candidate's present health, his own past history or a family history of epilepsy (Grand Mal) or minor seizures (Petit Mal).

It is the Medical Examiner's duty to ensure that the candidate's **Cardiovascular System,** which will include heart function and blood pressure, is satisfactory and performs within defined limits. The **Electro-Cardiogram** (ECG) is used to record electrical changes within the heart muscle and can be used to diagnose abnormalities. Under ordinary circumstances, this special investigation is not required when the candidate is under 40 years of age. **Cardiovascular Disease** is the commonest cause for Senior Air Line Transport Pilots being grounded for medical reasons. The community at large is very well aware of the incidence of sudden death due to **Coronary Thrombosis.** By using the ECG it is possible to detect early ischaemic changes in the heart muscle before the sufferer may be aware of any symptoms or before a coronary catastrophe could reasonably be expected to occur. Ischaemic changes in the heart muscle may be defined as areas of muscle damage due to lack of oxygen (**Hypoxia**) as a consequence of an impaired blood supply due to thickening of the arterial walls (**Arteriosclerosis**). A low blood pressure or more correctly a poor pulse pressure is sometimes associated with fainting attacks (**Syncope**). This state of affairs is more often encountered in lean, asthenic individuals and in people with a nervous or inadequate personality.

The **Respiratory System** must be demonstrated to be efficient for the proper interchange of oxygen and carbon dioxide, and past or present disease should be excluded by a chest X-ray.

Kidney function must be satisfactory and this is usually assessed by examination of a specimen of urine passed by the candidate in the presence of the examiner. It is customary to examine the urine for **Specific Gravity**, for this gives an indication of renal concentration, the presence of **Sugar** to exclude **Diabetes** and for **Protein** content to detect **Renal Damage**.

The **Ear, Nose** and **Throat** must be examined to ensure that the **Eustachian Tubes** are patent and afford a two-way flow of air; that the ear drums are healthy, and that hearing ability is within normal limits. The Student or Private Pilot's ability to hear is assessed as satisfactory if he can hear a whisper at a distance of twenty feet when he is facing away from the examiner. **Auditory Acuity** is more accurately measured by audiometry. For this purpose an audiometer is used and decibel (dB) loss is estimated at the following frequencies (cycles per second, now called hertz)—250, 500, 1000, 1500, 2000, 3000, 4000, 6000, and 8000.

It is hoped that, by reading this short review, the Private Pilot will appreciate the responsibilities which the Medical Assessor must accept and which he must discharge conscientiously in the interests of Flight Safety.

The Student Pilot will soon become aware of the enormous work load and concentration required of him during the initial stages of learning to fly. Slowly, by constant practice, he will begin to fly by instinct and when this facility has been acquired he will find more time to keep a good look-out whilst at the same time being able to conduct simple R/T procedures. Once he has gone solo and has settled down to basic flying with the use of radio, he will find himself able to navigate by map reading and ground reference. If he is a wise man, he will very soon appreciate the necessity for thorough and careful pre-flight planning in order to relieve himself of unnecessary tasks and avoidable anxieties whilst in the air. The acquisition of a Private Pilot's Licence may be a cause for celebration but it is no excuse to give up further training for, in order to fly safely many more skills are required, not the least of which will be the ability to fly accurately on instruments and in order to do just that, a basic understanding of aeromedicine is required. It is for this reason, above all others, that the author set himself the task of writing this book.

2. The Atmosphere and Respiration

1. The Atmosphere

The atmosphere, which weighs more than 5600 trillion tons, surrounds the earth to a depth of 500 miles and is prevented from escaping into space by the force of the earth's gravitational pull. The sun, which is 93 million miles away, is our source of energy, and together with our atmosphere, provides those .environmental conditions which are necessary for the existence of life on earth. Man, a very small terrestrial creature, is able to survive only in the lowest 20000 ft of this gaseous envelope.

The atmosphere, which consists mainly of **Oxygen** and **Nitrogen**, contains some **Water Vapour** and minute quantities of **Carbon Dioxide** and inert gases such as **Argon, Neon, Helium** and **Krypton.**

Water vapour is one of the invisible constituents of the air, as salt is one of the invisible constituents of sea water. Whilst the amount of water vapour which can be carried by a parcel of air will depend, to some extent, on barometric pressure, it is largely determined by atmospheric temperature. For instance, 1000 grammes (g) of air at 16°C can contain 11 g of water vapour. If the temperature should drop by 7°C, then 6 g of this water vapour will materialize as fine droplets to form cloud, or as larger droplets to cause drizzle or rain. One calorie of heat is required to raise one gramme of water through one degree centigrade, but nearly 600 calories of solar energy are needed before one gramme of water on the earth's surface can be transformed by evaporation into water vapour. At **Dew Point**, it is these calories which are released as latent heat when water vapour precipitates and cloud formation takes place. At night, under a clear sky, the earth's surface will cool rapidly by loss of heat through radiation but, when covered by a blanket of low-level cloud, it will behave like a teapot protected by a tea-cosy and stay warm. Thus water vapour which gives birth to cloud and helps to provide our weather by transporting huge quantities of water and heat over the surface of the earth possesses an importance out of all proportion to its tiny physical presence which constitutes only one per cent of our atmosphere up to 70 000 ft.

At sea level, the International Standard Atmosphere is defined as having a temperature of 15°C and a pressure of 760 mm of mercury. This pressure is often expressed as 14·7 pounds per square inch on a Diver's Equipment, 29·96 inches of mercury on a domestic barometer and as 1013·2 millibars (mb) on the subscale of an aircraft's altimeter. By definition, a millibar is a pressure of 1000 dynes per square centimetre . . . and if you want to know what a **Dyne** is . . . well, it is a unit of force which, acting for one second on a mass of one gramme, will give it a velocity of one centimetre per second!

It is perhaps appropriate to recognize here the fact that the United Kingdom is now changing to the SI metric system of units—a logical system with many potential advantages. In this system the unit of force is the *newton*—that force which produces an acceleration of one metre per second on a mass of one kilogramme, and the unit of pressure is the newton per square metre—physically quite a small quantity. The millibar is equal to 100 newtons per square metre.

The situation during this interim period is inevitably rather confusing, with a mixture of units from different systems in current use, particularly in aviation, and it is felt best to offer data in whichever form pilots are most likely to encounter during the next few years.

Dalton's Law states that the total pressure of a gaseous mixture is the sum total of the partial pressures exerted by each constituent and, because air consists of approximately 21 %

oxygen and 78 % nitrogen, it follows that the partial pressure of oxygen at sea level is $760 \times \frac{21}{100} = 160$ mm of mercury.

The physical properties of the atmosphere make it possible to divide it into layers around the earth, in a fashion similar to the whorls within an onion. The layer lowest in the atmosphere and nearest to the earth is called the **Troposphere**, which is separated by the **Tropopause** from the **Stratosphere** above. The tropopause, which varies in height from 25000 to 45000 ft, is highest over the Equator and lowest over the Poles.

An increase in altitude will bring about a decrease in pressure since there will be less weight of air above to be supported. Whilst a gas becomes hot if it is compressed, for example, pumping up your bicycle tyres, it follows that it cools when it expands, and for this reason lower temperatures will be encountered at higher altitudes. The rate at which air cools with increasing altitude due to expansion is called the **Adiabatic Lapse Rate** and the **International Standard Adiabatic Lapse Rate** is defined as 2°C per thousand feet. Temperatures of minus 45 to minus 80°C are encountered at the tropopause where they create a climatic paradox, for, since the tropopause is lower in these regions, it will be warmer over the Poles than over the Equator. In the Stratosphere above, temperature remains fairly constant.

Solar Energy (Insolation) passes through the atmosphere and heats the ground. The atmosphere itself is largely unaffected by the passage through it of radiant or solar energy, but is warmed from below by convective currents caused by radiation of heat from the earth's surface.

Table 1 shows the relationship between altitude and atmospheric pressure. It will be seen that atmospheric pressure decreases logarithmically with increasing altitude.

Under conditions of cloud formation the air below cloud which is rising will cool adiabatically at an approximate rate of 3°C per thousand feet (**Dry Adiabatic Lapse Rate**). Once dew point has been reached and cloud formation is taking place, the release of latent heat will retard the adiabatic rate of cooling to about 1·5°C per thousand feet (**Saturated Adiabatic Lapse Rate**).

Table 1

ATMOSPHERIC PRESSURE CHANGES ASSOCIATED WITH ALTITUDE

Altitude (ft)	Pressure (mm Mercury)	Altitude (ft)	Pressure (mm Mercury)
0	760·0	20000	349·1
500	746·4	21000	334·6
1000	732·9	22000	320·8
2000	706·6	23000	307·4
3000	681·1	24000	294·4
4000	656·3	25000	281·8
5000	632·3	26000	269·8
6000	609·0	27000	258·0
7000	586·4	28000	246·8
8000	564·4	29000	236·0
9000	543·2	30000	225·6
10000	522·6	31000	215·4
11000	502·6	32000	205·6
12000	483·3	33000	196·3
13000	464·4	34000	187·3
14000	446·4	35000	178·7
15000	428·8	36000	170·3
16000	411·8	37000	162·4
17000	395·3	38000	154·8
18000	379·4	39000	147·5
19000	364·0	40000	140·7

2. Respiration

Air enters the body through the nose, where it is filtered, warmed and humidified. By the act of inspiration it is drawn down the windpipe and conducted to the air sacs (**Alveoli**) in the lungs. Here, oxygen diffuses into the bloodstream by pressure gradient. The total surface area of all the alveoli, available for diffusion, is equivalent to the floor area of a room 36 ft long and 20 ft wide. Oxygen combines with haemoglobin to form oxyhaemoglobin in the red blood corpuscles, and is conveyed to all parts of the body. Under atmospheric pressure at sea level, 100 millilitres (ml) of blood will carry 19 millilitres of oxygen. One of the waste products of the body's biochemical reactions (**Metabolism**) is carbon dioxide, which is carried away in the blood stream. In the lungs, by pressure gradient, carbon dioxide diffuses across the alveolar membrane to enter the **Alveolar Air** from whence, by the act of expiration, it is expelled from the body. The respiratory centre in the brain stem, which controls the rate of respiration, is stimulated by increased amounts of carbon dioxide, dissolved in the blood to form carbonic acid. Increased amounts of carbonic acid in the blood will also increase the acidity of the body, whilst decreased amounts will tend to make the body more alkaline.

The total lung capacity is 5 litres (l), and at rest man needs to breathe in about 8 l of air per minute. Violent exercise will increase this requirement to as much as 60 litres per minute. At rest, each breath will involve the movement of about one half of a litre of air in and out of the lungs; a mere tenth of their capacity.

It follows that the lungs are far from being cleansed of their used air with each breath, and this state of affairs is further aggravated by the constant removal of oxygen from the alveolar air to the bloodstream, and the constant addition to the alveolar air of carbon dioxide from the bloodstream. Thus the composition of alveolar air is going to be very different from atmospheric air; alveolar air contains, in addition to nitrogen and oxygen, very significant amounts of water vapour and carbon dioxide. At sea level the partial pressure exerted by the water vapour content is 47 mm of mercury and that of carbon dioxide 40 mm of mercury, thus making the pressure of dry alveolar air 713 mm of mercury (760 minus 47 mm of mercury).

The composition of dry alveolar air is—

Oxygen .	.	.	.	.14·5%
Nitrogen	.	.	.	.80·0%
Carbon dioxide		.	.	. 5·5%

Therefore, at sea level, whereas atmospheric oxygen pressure is 160 mm of mercury, alveolar oxygen is reduced to 103 mm of mercury.

From Fig. 1 it will be seen that by climbing to 10000 ft a situation is created where, although the alveolar oxygen pressure

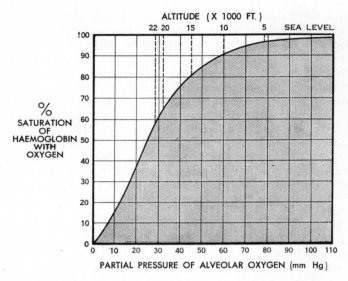

Fig. 1. Relationship between the Oxygen-carrying Capacity
of the Blood and the Partial Pressure of Alveolar Oxygen at
Various Altitudes

has dropped by 40 mm of mercury, the blood is still saturated to
90% of its capacity with oxygen. Trouble gets more serious
above 10000 ft, when relatively small decreases of alveolar
oxygen pressure are associated with disproportionately large
reductions in the oxygen carrying capacity of the blood. To sum
up, man can fly happily in the lowest 8000 ft of his atmosphere,
but at altitudes above 10000 ft his efficiency and then his life
are placed in jeopardy if supplementary oxygen is not provided.

3. Hypoxia

Man, who possesses no means by which he can store oxygen,
needs a constant and adequate supply to sustain his metabolism.
The brain, nervous pathways, and sensory organs (the central
nervous system) are particularly sensitive to lack of oxygen;

which is called hypoxia. The term hypoxia, which will be used throughout this book, is often confused with **Anoxia**, which really means a total absence of oxygen.

Dr. Paul Bert, a Frenchman, was in the forefront of research into aviation medicine and was the first to investigate the effects of hypoxia. In 1875 he was able to describe human reactions to hypoxia from experiments he conducted by producing low atmospheric pressures in a decompression chamber. In the same year three of his associaties ascended to 28000 ft in a balloon and only one, Monsieur Tissandier, survived the ordeal and lived to describe most graphically the symptoms and signs of hypoxia. His words are as true to-day as they were nearly 100 years ago—

"I now come to the fateful moments when we were overcome by the terrific action of reduced pressure. At 22,900 feet . . . torpor had seized me. I write nevertheless . . . though I have no clear recollection of writing. We are rising, at 24,000 feet the condition of torpor that overcomes me is extraordinary. Body and mind become feebler . . . there is no suffering. On the contrary one feels an inward joy. There is no thought of the dangerous position; one rises and is glad to be rising. I soon felt myself so weak that I could not turn my head to look at my companions . . . I wished to call out that we were now at 26,000 feet, but my tongue was paralysed. All at once I fell down powerless and lost all further memory."

A more recent but equally dramatic account of hypoxia was provided by the navigator of a Halifax bomber after returning from a bombing mission over Europe in the Second World War. The aircraft had been flying at altitudes which varied between 18000 and 24000 ft and for a period of two hours the pilot had suffered from hypoxia, due to a failure of his oxygen supply whilst at an altitude of 20000 ft. The navigator wrote—

"The captain became very talkative but resented any suggestions that he was behaving abnormally. On seeing the marker flares over the target, he found he could not take his eyes off them and forced the aircraft into a steep dive. Afterwards, he said that he could only read the larger figures on the instrument panel and these appeared far away. When he realised the aircraft was out of control the engineer trimmed the aircraft. The pilot resented this and assaulted the engineer. He then gave the order to bale out, which we cancelled. He opened the window to look out, and was only prevented from falling out by the engineer, who hauled him in. He said that he felt very happy, and had no feeling of fear even when he tried to force land on a cloud, thinking he was near the ground. On one occasion he informed us that we were below ground. After being forced to take oxygen from the spare helmet and mask he gradually recovered his senses and was able to fly the required course to base, although he suffered from headache which persisted after landing."

Even as low as 4000 ft night vision begins to fail, and it becomes increasingly difficult to distinguish dimly-lit objects in the cockpit, in the air, and on the ground. At 8000 ft mental acuity is reduced, whilst at heights above 10000 ft impaired judgment becomes apparent to an observer. The symptoms and signs of hypoxia are many and varied but will include a reduced awareness to surrounding conditions, a failure to appreciate danger, an euphoric acceptance that all is well when in fact disaster may be at hand, and mood swings which permit depression to give way to hilarity and lead either to physical violence or drowsiness; a state not dissimilar to that of the drunk who may decide to fight it out, or drop comatosed across the back of a chair. Hypoxia may cause giddiness, light-headedness and headaches, and the lips, fingers, and toes may become blue through a failure on the part of the circulation to maintain a sufficient supply of well oxygenated blood to the peripheral parts of the body. Further degrees of hypoxia will cause muscular spasms, inco-ordinated movements of the arms and legs, visual and auditory failure, semi-consciousness and, finally, unconsciousness. Whilst the state of hypoxia is becoming established the aviator may remain unaware of any symptoms of breathlessness and pass from euphoria into unconsciousness without realizing that anything is amiss.

Increased susceptibility to hypoxia is caused by—

COLD   Remember that at 10 000 ft the outside temperature is likely to be minus 5°C.

FATIGUE   Prolonged instrument flying in cloud may cause marked mental weariness.

ALCOHOL   Do not drink and fly; fly first and drink later.

DRUGS   Do not take motion sickness pills; many of them are mental sedatives. "Cold cures" have the same effect. (*See* Ch. 5.) Do not take amphetamines such as Dexedrine or Benzedrine to keep awake. These drugs reduce your awareness to danger and, when their effect has worn off, dizziness and headaches can give rise to mental confusion. (*See* Ch. 5.)

SMOKING   Carbon monoxide in tobacco smoke combines with the haemoglobin in the red blood corpuscles to form **Carboxyhaemoglobin** and reduces the oxygen carrying capacity of the blood. It is possible for a heavy smoker to have an inbuilt biological altimeter which reads 8000 ft when he is on the ground.

OBESITY   If you are overweight, watch your calories and go on a high protein diet.

4. Hyperventilation

This is a state of over-breathing brought about by fear, excitement, or anxiety. Its symptoms may be indistinguishable from those of hypoxia, and if at altitude you should feel that you are suffering from either hypoxia or hyperventilation carry out the following checks—

(*a*) check the **Contents Gauge** on the oxygen supply,

(*b*) check the **Flow Meter,**

(*c*) check your oxygen pipe line; it may have become disconnected,

(*d*) check for **Leaks** around your face mask.

ACTION TO BE TAKEN

If there is anything wrong with the oxygen supply which cannot be corrected immediately, descend to a safe altitude as quickly as possible. If there is nothing wrong with the oxygen supply; compose yourself, for you are suffering from hyperventilation and not hypoxia. Hyperventilation, which has been caused by over-breathing, has washed nearly all the carbon dioxide out of your body, and biochemically you have become too alkaline. It is this degree of alkalinity which has caused your symptoms; symptoms which will cease as soon as you stop over-breathing and allow the carbon dioxide content of the blood to return to normal. Therefore make a conscious effort to breathe gently and slowly.

5. Environmental Temperatures

The light aircraft pilot, with his heated cabin and comparatively low service ceiling, is unlikely to fall victim to exposure unless he survives a crash in mountainous terrain. But the glider pilot, without cabin heat, and in a high-performance aircraft capable of using lift to 40000 ft or more, is particularly prone to this danger which may lead to low-temperature feebleness **(Hypothermia)** or be responsible for icing up of unsuitable oxygen equipment.

Factors which tend to raise cockpit temperatures above those of the outside air are—

FRICTIONAL KINETIC ENERGY induced by the aircraft's passage through the air. This source of heat is only of significance in high-speed flight and is given by the formula

$$T = 0.85 \times \frac{(V)^2}{(100)}$$

where T = temperature rise in degrees centigrade.
V = indicated air speed.

SOLAR ENERGY which produces the "greenhouse" effect is of much great importance to the light aircraft and glider pilot. Short-wave solar heat radiation which passes through the aircraft's transparencies is re-radiated and trapped within the cockpit as long-wave heat radiation.

Table 2
AMBIENT.AIR TEMPERATURE AND ALTITUDE

Altitude (ft)	Temperature (°C)
sea level	15
5000	5
10000	− 5
15000	−15
20000	−24
25000	−34
30000	−45
35000	−55
40000	−55 or more depending on height of tropopause

Table 2 shows temperatures likely to be encountered at various altitudes. Loss of body heat due to low environmental temperatures will depend on—

(a) The absolute temperature.
(b) The volume of air passing over the body. This will depend on the velocity of the air current and the duration of exposure.
(c) Efficiency of protective clothing.

Frostbite is one example of tissue damage caused by cold which may be experienced by glider pilots whilst soaring in mountain waves to heights where the ambient air temperature can be as low as $-50°C$. The effect of such low temperature is, initially, to reduce the rate of flow of blood in the surface blood vessels and to cause the skin to blanch, the flesh to become hard, and the affected parts to become numb. Frostbite most commonly attacks the fingers and toes, but the face and ears may also be involved. Under these conditions tissue damage is likely to be the result of exposure to extreme cold for a relatively short period of time (20–30 min). Sudden loss of the aircraft's canopy may cause extensive damage to the skin of the face and result in blisters similar to those associated with second-degree burns due to heat. All cases of frostbite require expert medical attention and the modern concept of treatment involves rapid re-warming of the affected tissues whilst transport to hospital is being arranged. The affected parts should be immersed in water at temperatures between 42 and $45°C$. If warm water is not obtainable, and no other source of heat available, the affected parts should be warmed under the armpits or in the groin.

Protection against frostbite may be afforded by suitable clothing which provides adequate thermal insulation. Since air is a poor thermal conductor, the body should be covered by several layers of clothing each of which should, in turn, enclose a sandwich-like layer of captive air. Woollen clothing, which is porous to sweat, should be worn next to the skin, for, should a layer of perspiration form around the body, insulation will break down due to the high thermal conductivity of water. The head and ears should be covered by a flying helmet and the face protected by a mask to which is attached the oxygen supply. Hypoxia will make the pilot even more prone to frostbite. The hands should be protected by two or more pairs of dry woollen gloves which cover the wrists but allow free movement of the fingers. Fleece-lined boots, specially warmed and dried, should be worn and should be big enough to allow free movement of the toes. The feet should be enclosed within several pairs of woollen stockings which have been specially dried and warmed for the occasion. Finally, if the ground is wet, the pilot should be carried out to the glider to avoid any possibility of his boots becoming covered with an outside layer of moisture.

6. Decompression Sickness

This condition is due to nitrogen dissolved in the tissue fluids bubbling out in gaseous form under reduced atmospheric pressure, in a manner similar to bubble formation in a soda-water syphon when the top is opened and the pressure allowed to drop. This condition, which is not likely to occur below 25000 ft, but has occurred at 14000 ft, will be affected by the duration of exposure to reduced atmospheric pressure. Symptoms vary with the amount of bubble formation and the tissues involved. Joint spaces and muscles are usually affected first, giving rise to stiffness in the joints and rheumatic-like pains in the muscles. If the chest organs are involved, the unfortunate victim will suffer from a painful choking sensation. Should bubbles form within the substance of the spinal cord or brain, then tingling sensations **(Parathesiae)** or paralysis, either temporary or permanent, may ensue.

CONDITIONS LIKELY TO INCREASE SUSCEPTIBILITY TO DECOMPRESSION SICKNESS

AGE — There is clear evidence to show that there is increasing susceptibility to decompression sickness with advancing years. It appears that susceptibility increases steadily with increasing age and that there is a noteworthy increase even at the lower end of the scale (age groups 17–25).

OBESITY — Evidence clearly shows that obesity increases susceptibility to decompression sickness and pilots of aircraft capable of high-altitude climbs should not allow their body weight to exceed 15 per cent of the average age/height/weight figures which appear in Tables 3 and 4. A further list of recommended weights is included in Table 5, for those interested in longevity.

Table 3
AVERAGE AGE/HEIGHT/WEIGHT FOR MEN

Average weights in pounds and kilogrammes
(in indoor clothing)

Height (in 1-inch heels)			17–19 years		20–24 years		25–29 years		30–39 years		40–49 years		50–59 years	
ft	in	cm	lb	kg	lb	kg	lb	kg	lb	kg	lb	kg	lb	kg
5	0	152.4	113	51.3	122	55.3	128	58.1	131	59.4	134	60.8	136	61.7
5	0½	153.7	114.5	51.9	123.5	56	129.5	58.7	132.5	60.1	135.5	61.5	137.5	62.4
5	1	154.9	116	52.6	125	56.7	131	59.4	134	60.8	137	62.1	139	63
5	1½	156.2	117.5	53.3	126.5	57.4	132.5	60.1	135.5	61.5	138.5	62.8	140.5	63.7
5	2	157.5	119	54	128	58.1	134	60.8	137	62.1	140	63.5	142	64.4
5	2½	158.8	121	54.9	130	59	136	61.7	139	63	142	64.4	143.5	65.1
5	3	160	123	55.8	132	59.9	138	62.6	141	64	144	65.3	145	65.8
5	3½	161.3	125	56.7	134	60.8	139.5	63.3	143	64.9	146	66.2	147	66.7
5	4	162.6	127	57.6	136	61.7	141	64	145	65.8	148	67.1	149	67.6
5	4½	163.8	129	58.5	137.5	62.4	142.5	64.6	147	66.7	150	68	151	68.5
5	5	165.1	131	59.4	139	63	144	65.3	149	67.6	152	68.9	153	69.4
5	5½	166.4	133	60.3	140.5	63.7	146	66.2	151	68.5	154	69.9	155	70.3
5	6	167.6	135	61.2	142	64.4	148	67.1	153	69.4	156	70.8	157	71.2
5	6½	168.9	137	62.1	143.5	65.1	149.5	67.8	155	70.3	158.5	71.9	159.5	72.3
5	7	170.2	139	63	145	65.8	151	68.5	157	71.2	161	73	162	73.5
5	7½	171.5	141	64	147	66.7	153	69.4	159	72.1	163	73.9	164	74.4
5	8	172.7	143	64.9	149	67.6	155	70.3	161	73	165	74.8	166	75.3
5	8½	174	145	65.8	151	68.5	157	71.2	163	73.9	167	75.6	168	76.2
5	9	175.3	147	66.7	153	69.4	159	72.1	165	74.8	169	76.7	170	77.1
5	9½	176.5	149	67.6	155	70.3	161	73	167.5	76	171.5	77.8	172.5	78.2
5	10	177.8	151	68.5	157	71.2	163	73.9	170	77.1	174	78.9	175	79.4
5	10½	179.1	153	69.4	159	72.1	165	74.8	172	78	176	79.8	177.5	80.5
5	11	180.3	155	70.3	161	73	167	75.8	174	78.9	178	80.8	180	81.6
5	11½	181.6	157.5	71.4	163.5	74.2	169.5	76.9	176.5	80.1	180.5	81.9	182.5	82.8
6	0	182.9	160	72.6	166	75.3	172	78	179	81.2	183	83	185	83.9
6	0½	184.2	162	73.5	168	76.2	174.5	79.2	181	82.1	185	83.9	187	84.8
6	1	185.4	164	74.4	170	77.1	177	80.3	183	83	187	84.8	189	85.7
6	1½	186.7	166	75.3	172	78	179.5	81.4	185.5	84.1	189.5	86	191.5	86.9
6	2	188	168	76.2	174	78.9	182	82.6	188	85.3	192	87.1	194	88
6	2½	189.2	170	77.1	176	79.8	184	83.5	190.5	86.4	194.5	88.2	196.5	89.1
6	3	190.5	172	78	178	80.8	186	84.4	193	87.5	197	89.4	199	90.3
6	3½	191.8	174	78.9	179.5	81.4	188	85.3	196	88.9	200	90.7	202	91.6
6	4	193	176	79.8	181	82.1	190	86.2	199	90.3	203	92.1	205	93

Table 4
AVERAGE AGE/HEIGHT/WEIGHT FOR WOMEN

Average weights in pounds and kilogrammes (in indoor clothing)

Height (in 2-inch heels)			17–19 years		20–24 years		25–29 years		30–39 years		40–49 years		50–59 years	
ft	in	cm	lb	kg	lb	kg	lb	kg	lb	kg	lb	kg	lb	kg
4	10	147·3	99	44·9	102	46·3	107	48·5	115	52·2	122	55·3	125	56·7
4	10½	148·6	100·5	45·6	103·5	46·9	108·5	49·2	116	52·6	123	55·8	126	57·2
4	11	149·9	102	46·3	105	47·6	110	49·9	117	53·1	124	56·2	127	57·6
4	11½	151·1	103·5	46·9	106·5	48·3	111·5	50·6	118·5	53·8	125·5	56·9	128·5	58·3
5	0	152·4	105	47·6	108	49	113	51·3	120	54·4	127	57·6	130	59
5	0½	153·7	107	48·5	110	49·9	114·5	51·9	121·5	55·1	128·5	58·3	131·5	59·6
5	1	154·9	109	49·4	112	50·8	116	52·6	123	55·8	130	59	133	60·3
5	1½	156·2	111	50·3	113·5	51·5	117·5	53·3	124·5	56·5	131·5	59·6	134·5	61
5	2	157·5	113	51·3	115	52·2	119	54	126	57·2	133	60·3	136	61·7
5	2½	158·8	114·5	51·9	116·5	52·8	120·5	54·7	127·5	57·8	134·5	61	138	62·6
5	3	160	116	52·6	118	53·5	122	55·3	129	58·5	136	61·7	140	63·5
5	3½	161·3	118	53·5	119·5	54·2	123·5	56	130·5	59·2	138	62·6	142	64·4
5	4	162·6	120	54·4	121	54·9	125	56·7	132	59·9	140	63·5	144	65·3
5	4½	163·8	122	55·3	123	55·8	127	57·6	133·5	60·6	141·5	64·2	146	66·2
5	5	165·1	124	56·2	125	56·7	129	58·5	135	61·2	143	64·9	148	67·1
5	5½	166·4	125·5	56·9	127	57·6	131	59·4	137	62·1	145	65·8	150	68
5	6	167·6	127	57·6	129	58·5	133	60·3	139	63	147	66·7	152	68·9
5	6½	168·9	128·5	58·3	130·5	59·2	134·5	61	140·5	63·7	149	67·6	154	69·9
5	7	170·2	130	59	132	59·9	136	61·7	142	64·4	151	68·5	156	70·8
5	7½	171·5	132	59·9	134	60·8	138	62·6	144	65·3	153	69·4	158	71·7
5	8	172·7	134	60·8	136	61·7	140	63·5	146	66·2	155	70·3	160	72·6
5	8½	174	136	61·7	138	62·6	142	64·4	148	67·1	157	71·2	162	73·5
5	9	175·3	138	62·6	140	63·5	144	65·3	150	68	159	72·1	164	74·4
5	9½	176·5	140	63·5	142	64·4	146	66·2	152	68·9	161·5	73·3	166·5	75·5
5	10	177·8	142	64·5	144	65·3	148	67·1	154	69·9	164	74·4	169	76·7
5	10½	179·1	144·5	65·5	146·5	66·5	150·5	68·3	156·6	71	166·5	75·5	171·5	77·8
5	11	180·3	147	66·7	149	67·6	153	69·4	159	72·1	169	76·7	174	78·9
5	11½	181·6	149·5	67·8	151·5	68·7	155·5	70·5	161·5	73·3	171·5	77·8	177	80·3
6	0	182·9	152	68·9	154	69·9	158	71·7	164	74·4	174	78·9	180	81·6

Table 5
RECOMMENDED WEIGHTS

Desirable weight in pounds and kilogrammes (in indoor clothing), ages 25 and over

Height (in shoes) ft in	cm	Small frame lb	Small frame kg	Medium frame lb	Medium frame kg	Large frame lb	Large frame kg
MEN							
5 2	157·5	112–120	50·8–54·4	118–129	53·5–58·5	126–141	57·2–64
5 3	160	115–123	52·2–55·8	121–133	54·9–60·3	129–144	58·5–65·5
5 4	162·6	118–126	53·5–57·2	124–136	56·2–61·7	132–148	59·9–67·1
5 5	165·1	121–129	54·9–58·5	127–139	57·6–63	135–152	61·2–68·9
5 6	167·6	124–133	56·2–60·3	130–143	59–64·9	138–156	62·6–70·8
5 7	170·2	128–137	58·1–62·1	134–147	60·8–66·7	142–161	64·4–73
5 8	172·7	132–141	59·9–64	138–152	62·6–68·9	147–166	66·7–75·3
5 9	175·3	136–145	61·7–65·8	142–156	64·4–70·8	151–170	68·5–77·1
5 10	177·8	140–150	63·5–68	146–160	66·2–72·6	155–174	70·3–78·9
5 11	180·3	144–154	65·3–69·9	150–165	68–74·8	159–179	72·1–81·2
6 0	182·9	148–158	67·1–71·7	154–170	69·9–77·1	164–184	74·4–83·5
6 1	185·4	152–162	68·9–73·5	158–175	71·7–79·4	168–189	76·2–85·7
6 2	188	156–167	70·8–75·7	162–180	73·5–81·6	173–194	78·5–88
6 3	190·5	160–171	72·6–77·6	167–185	75·7–83·5	178–199	80·7–90·3
6 4	193	164–175	74·4–79·4	172–190	78·1–86·2	182–204	82·7–92·5
WOMEN							
4 10	147·3	92–98	41·7–44·5	96–107	43·5–48·5	104–119	47·2–54
4 11	149·9	94–101	42·6–45·8	98–110	44·5–49·9	106–122	48·1–55·3
5 0	152·4	96–104	43·5–47·2	101–113	45·8–51·3	109–125	49·4–56·7
5 1	154·9	99–107	44·9–48·5	104–116	47·2–52·5	112–128	50·8–58·1
5 2	157·5	102–110	46·3–49·9	107–119	48·5–54	115–131	52·2–59·4
5 3	160	105–113	47·6–51·3	110–122	49·9–55·3	118–134	53·5–60·8
5 4	162·6	108–116	49–52·6	113–126	51·3–57·2	121–138	54·9–62·6
5 5	165·1	111–119	50·3–54	116–130	52·6–59	125–142	56·7–64·4
5 6	167·6	114–123	51·7–55·8	120–135	54·4–61·2	129–146	58·5–66·2
5 7	170·2	118–127	53·5–57·6	124–139	56·2–63	133–150	60·3–68
5 8	172·7	122–131	55·3–59·4	128–143	58·1–64·9	137–154	62·1–69·9
5 9	175·3	126–135	57·2–61·2	132–147	59·9–66·7	141–158	64–71·7
5 10	177·8	130–140	59–63·5	136–151	61·7–68·5	145–163	65·8–73·9
5 11	180·3	134–144	60·8–65·3	140–155	63·5–70·3	149–168	67·6–76·2
6 0	182·9	138–148	·62·6–67·1	144–159	65·3–72·1	153–173	69·4–78·5

RATE OF CLIMB — Rapid rates of climb should be avoided in unpressurized aircraft.

EXERCISE — Exercise has a profound effect upon susceptibility to decompression sickness, those parts most involved in exercise being the most likely sites for symptoms. This explains why the shoulder and upper arm muscles and their associated joint spaces are the sites most commonly associated with symptoms caused by this condition.

FATIGUE — Go to bed early the night before you intend to gain the World Height Record in a glider.

ALCOHOL — Twelve hours should separate bottle from throttle.

RE-EXPOSURE — Re-exposure to decompression, within a 24-hr period will lead to increased susceptibility to decompression sickness. It is generally agreed that 48 hrs should separate further exposure to the dangers of this serious condition.

SUB-AQUA DIVING AND FLYING — It is unwise to fly within 48 hrs of sub-aqua diving to depths greater than 33 ft (two atmospheres absolute), for the reduced partial pressure of nitrogen associated with altitude will increase susceptibility to decompression sickness. This danger is well known to professional crews in Civil Aviation who may well be tempted to enjoy this exciting sport whilst resting at route staging posts. According to the Flight Level being flown, most civilian airliners maintain a cabin pressure of 5000 to 8000 ft equivalent (632 to 565 mm Hg). The author, as a member of the Royal National Life

Boat Institution, has been concerned in recent years with the immediate treatment of the "bends" among professional shell-fish divers working off the northwest coast of Cornwall. These seriously ill men must be transported some 80 miles to Plymouth for treatment in hyperbaric chambers operated by the Royal Navy at their Diving School in Devonport. As speed is essential, many are transported by Royal Navy S.A.R. (Search and Rescue) helicopters and great care is exercised by flying as low as is compatible with safety, to ensure that their already serious condition is not further aggravated by the harmful effects of altitude.

ACTION TO BE TAKEN TO REDUCE THE POSSIBILITY OF DECOMPRESSION SICKNESS

If soaring in mountain wave conditions it is wise to pre-breathe pure oxygen from take-off level in order to wash out as much nitrogen as possible from the blood.

TREATMENT OF DECOMPRESSION SICKNESS

Minor joint pains usually disappear if descent to a lower altitude is made; here, the increased atmospheric pressure will cause gaseous nitrogen to dissove back into the tissue fluids. If symptoms persist after landing, or occur within 24 hrs of a high altitude flight, a doctor must be called at once and the patient removed to a hospital equipped with a compression chamber. The prevention and treatment of decompression sickness **must** be taken seriously, for death may follow apparently trivial episodes.

7. Oxygen Systems Suitable for Light Aircraft and Gliders

Oxygen systems fitted as an integral part of an aircraft's equipment consist of the following component parts—

(*a*) Oxygen suitable for breathing.

(*b*) Oxygen storage container.

(*c*) Regulator.

(*d*) Face mask.

(*e*) High-pressure tubing to conduct oxygen from the storage cylinder to the regulator.

(*f*) Low-pressure tubing to conduct oxygen from the regulator to the face mask.

OXYGEN SUITABLE FOR BREATHING. This must conform to the following requirements—

(*a*) Free from odour.

(*b*) Not less than 98·5% pure.

(*c*) Free from any toxic substances, such as degreasing agents.

(*d*) Contain not more than 0·002% of carbon monoxide.

(*e*) A sample of oxygen drawn from a cylinder charged to between 1600 and 2000 lb per sq. in. must not contain more than 0·02 g of water per cubic metre (standard temperature and pressure) as measured by means of a high-pressure hygrometer of approved type.

OXYGEN STORAGE CONTAINER

Oxygen is stored at a pressure of 1800 lb per sq. in. in steel containers of varying capacities.

OXYGEN SYSTEMS IN CURRENT USE FOR HEIGHTS NOT EXCEEDING 40000 FT

The earliest form of oxygen supply was very simple and gave a continuous flow of oxygen. Since the act of inspiration occupies only two-fifths of the time taken to complete a respiratory cycle, this system proved most wasteful and has been discarded. It has been superseded by two systems which differ fundamentally both in design and application. These two systems, called respectively the **Economiser system** and the **Oxygen Demand System**, are now described in detail.

THE ECONOMISER SYSTEM

THE REGULATOR. The function of the regulator, which incorporates a reduction valve, is to accept oxygen from the storage container, reduce its pressure, and pass it on at a suitable rate of flow to the user. Design features of this regulator include—

(a) An "On" and "Off" selector switch.
(b) An oxygen contents gauge.
(c) Oxygen flow selector switch for **"Normal"** or **"High"** Flow.
(d) Two flow indicators.

The rate of oxygen flow is indicated only as far as the regulator, and therefore does not register the actual flow of oxygen from the regulator to the user. Thus, in the economizer system, it is essential for the user to feel puffs of oxygen coming into the mask before he can be assured that he is receiving a supply of oxygen. Pre-flight checks must include a **"Puff Check"**. This check should be done before the engine is started, and it is worth knowing that the flow of oxygen into the mask is more easily felt if the mask is held over the eyes for this check.

THE ECONOMIZER UNIT. This unit is fitted on the low-pressure side of the system and is placed between the regulator and the mask. It is designed to convert the continuous flow of oxygen delivered by the regulator to an intermittent flow before it is delivered to the mask. The economizer consists essentially of an inflatable bag, into which oxygen flows from the regulator. The out-flow from the bag to the mask is governed by a trip valve. During expiration the trip valve closes and oxygen, which would otherwise flow to waste, fills the bag. During inspiration, the trip valve lifts and the bag deflates, discharging its oxygen content into the mask. The economizer unit doubles the endurance from a single cylinder of oxygen.

THE MASK. The mask, which may incorporate a microphone, is fitted with expiratory valves and an inlet or "cheek" valve. The cheek valve allows the controlled dilution of oxygen to take place when the **"Normal"** rate of oxygen flow is selected;

for this valve is, in effect, a lightly loaded inlet valve. During inspiration, oxygen flows into the mask from the economizer bag until this is deflated. If, at this stage, the act of inspiration is continued, suction will cause the cheek valve to open and allow air to pass into the mask; the user will breathe this air, as well as a small but continuous flow of oxygen, through the open trip valve from the economizer bag. When the **"High"** rate of oxygen flow is selected the economizer bag never fully deflates and the cheek valve does not open; thus there is no controlled air dilution of the oxygen supply, and in effect, a continuous flow of oxygen is established—which is most wasteful and will reduce the endurance of the available oxygen supply.

Although the economizer system is simple, reliable, inexpensive, and comfortable to wear, it has a limited capability and three main disadvantages, namely—

(*a*) It does not allow for changing rates of respiration.
(*b*) It does not give any indication of function other than the information that oxygen is flowing through the regulator at the "Normal" or "High" rate.
(*c*) It is unsuitable if pressure breathing is required.

OXYGEN DEMAND SYSTEM (DILUTER DEMAND SYSTEM)

This system will provide either pure oxygen or a mixture of oxygen and air, barometrically controlled, on demand by the user and at a pressure of 2 mm of mercury above ambient pressure in either a pressurized or unpressurized cabin.

OXYGEN STORAGE CONTAINER. In most cases this will be similar to that already described, but with the introduction of liquid oxygen containers a more sophisticated unit can now be installed.

THE REGULATOR. This type of regulator will reduce the storage pressure of oxygen, and deliver a flow of oxygen through a wide-bore flexible tube to the mask during active inspiration on the part of the user.

AIRMIX OR DILUTER UNIT. Pure oxygen is only essential at altitudes in excess of 30000 ft. Air, increasingly enriched by oxygen, is sufficient between 10000 and 30000 ft. The oxygen demand system is usually modified so that air can be mixed with oxygen in correct proportions depending on cabin pressure in the aircraft at any height up to 30000 ft. At this altitude the **Airmix Orifice** closes completely and allows only pure oxygen to be supplied to the user. This unit contains three design features—

- (*a*) An expanding barometric capsule which accurately controls the oxygen/air mixture.
- (*b*) A non-return valve which prevents the loss of oxygen.
- (*c*) The **Airmix Unit** can be removed from the circuit by a selector lever, should 100% oxygen be required for any reason below 30000 ft.

SAFETY PRESSURE. The regulator in this system incorporates a safety factor by providing a supply of oxygen or oxygen/air mixture to the mask at a pressure of 2 mm of mercury above ambient cabin pressure. This safety pressure is created by adding a spring loading to the diaphragm which opens the demand valve. Thus, in order for this valve to close and stop any further flow from the regulator, the pressure within the mask must rise to a pressure of 2 mm of mercury higher than the ambient cabin pressure. When the user draws a breath, the pressure within the mask falls below **Ambient +2 mm of Mercury** and initiates a flow from the regulator at a stage when the pressure within the mask is still above ambient cabin pressure; this does not affect comfort but makes certain that any leak will be outward and not inward.

INDICATION OF OXYGEN FLOW. Each act of inspiration by the user causes a flow of oxygen from the regulator to the mask and initiates a pictorial indication of its flow by a movement of the **"Doll's Eye"**, which shows white. Even if the oxygen supply is turned off or is exhausted, it is still possible to breathe through the regulator providing "Normal" oxygen flow has been selected by the lever, but only up to an altitude of 30000 ft when, as already stated, the Airmix Unit stops the flow of air into the system. The "Doll's Eye" will not operate unless oxygen is flowing into the system, and if the "Doll's Eye" remains either **Black** or **White** there is something wrong with the system.

OXYGEN DEMAND MASK. Since the regulator has been designed to supply oxygen or oxygen/air mixture under pressure it follows that the mask must be capable of holding that pressure. For this requirement to be met, the following two design features have been incorporated in the demand mask

Mask Seal. The mask must be capable of fitting snugly on the face to prevent loss outwards or any leak inwards of ambient air. In order to achieve this the rubber at the perimeter of the mask as it approaches the face doubles back on itself in a gentle curve for a short way. Thus the same surface which is the outside of the mask is also the surface in close contact with the skin. As the pressure builds up on the inside of the mask, it not only forces the front of the mask outwards, but also presses the reflected edge more firmly on to the face. The provision of a toggle harness permits the mask to be clamped more firmly on the face when a high-pressure seal is required in an emergency.

Compensated Expiratory Valve. This valve is designed so that the pressure in the mask inlet tube is applied to the under-surface of the expiratory valve by a compensating tube. As oxygen is delivered by the regulator under pressure it creates a force within the mask which tends to open the expiratory valve, but by way of the compensating tube an equal force is applied to the under-surface of this valve so that it remains closed, and the pressure in the mask is able to rise.

CHOICE OF SYSTEMS

Both the economizer and oxygen demand systems are very satisfactory for use within the heated cabin of any light aircraft with a service ceiling of 30000 ft. Since the economizer system is more simple, less expensive, and easier to maintain, it remains the system of choice for most light aircraft owners.

For glider pilots and owners of light aircraft without cabin heat and a service ceiling of 40000 ft, much more serious problems could arise which make the provision of some sort of oxygen demand system essential. I refer to the danger of failure of the economizer system due to low environmental temperatures, for it must be clearly understood that—

    (*a*) **Expired alveolar air** is fully saturated with water vapour.
    (*b*) Ambient air temperature at 10 000 ft is likely to be $-5°C$.

The face mask which is suitable for use with the economizer system allows air to enter through the cheek valve and affords little protection against leaks either outwards or inwards around the area where the face mask comes in contact with the skin. Water vapour in expired air quickly condenses in the presence of only a small drop in temperature (a physical property used to advantage by many people to clean their spectacles). If water vapour should condense and freeze within the mask, free movement of the trip valve may be affected; indeed it may seize up altogether and prevent any flow of oxygen or allow a continuous flow of oxygen which could quickly exhaust the supply within the cylinder. In either case hypoxia may overcome the pilot before he can descend to a safe altitude. This danger must be clearly understood by every glider pilot before attempting a high-altitude climb in wave or cumulo-nimbus cloud formation when using the economizer system.

8. Essential Facts to Remember

    1. Air may be breathed safely at ambient pressure up to an altitude of 8000 ft.
    2. Pure oxygen, or a mixture of air increasingly enriched by oxygen, will be required at altitudes between 10 000 and 30 000 ft. The average person needs between 8 and 10 l per min. Physical activity and mental anxiety will increase the volume required. Fat people need more than thin people.
    3. Pure oxygen will be required at altitudes between 30 000 and 40 000 ft.
    4. Above 40 000 ft special pressure-breathing oxygen equipment must be used to maintain efficiency.
    5. Pure oxygen will maintain sea-level conditions up to 34 000 ft.

6. Pure oxygen at 40000 ft will give an alveolar oxygen pressure similar to breathing air at 10000 ft.
7. Any air leaks into the oxygen supply or mask above 25000 ft will cause hypoxia. Unconsciousness may occur should the oxygen supply fail at any altitude above 14000 ft and may occur within a minute at 30000 ft.
8. Times of useful consciousness following a failure in oxygen supply will vary from individual to individual and will depend on the amount of activity involved (*see* Table 6).

Table 6
TIMES OF USEFUL CONSCIOUSNESS FOLLOWING FAILURE
OF OXYGEN SUPPLY AT VARIOUS ALTITUDES

Altitude (ft) above sea level	Sudden Failure of Oxygen Supply	
	moderate activity	minimal activity
22000	5 minutes	10 minutes
25000	2 ,,	3 ,,
28000	1 ,,	1½ ,,
30000	45 seconds	1¼ ,,
35000	30 ,,	45 seconds
40000	12 ,,	15 ,,

9. Never forget that oxygen is used to prevent hypoxia. Select oxygen or controlled oxygen/air mixture at an altitude between 8000 and 10000 ft and remember that at 10000 ft failing mental faculties are apparent to an observer. Don't take risks; for if you do, you may not live to find out why you died!!
10. Make regular routine checks of your oxygen system every few minutes even if you feel perfectly fit and well.
11. Decompression sickness is a dangerous condition which can be caused by high-altitude climbs in unpressurized aircraft; it is most serious and requires expert medical

attention. Pre-breathing pure oxygen from take-off may help to prevent this condition.

12. Oxygen Systems

  (i) *Aircraft with cabin heat and a service ceiling of 30 000 ft.* The economizer system is the cheapest and meets all requirements.

  (ii) *Aircraft without cabin heat and a service ceiling of 40 000 ft.* The oxygen demand system should be used for the reasons already stated. If all high-altitude climbs could be done in clear air during summer time, the solar "greenhouse" effect would probably protect you from hypoxia up to 30 000 ft by preventing a failure of the economizer system through freezing.

3. The Eye and Vision

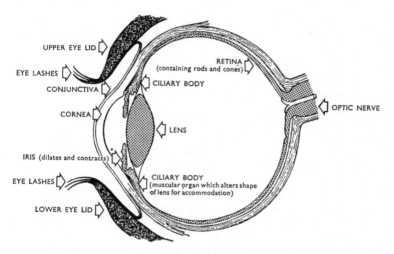

FIG. 2. The Human Eye

1. The Eye

Electromagnetic waves within the visual spectrum enter the eye through the cornea and are focused by the lens on the retina. Here, nerve endings interpret the impulses and transmit them, via the optic nerve, to the brain where an image is brought to conscious level. Sensory endings in the retina consist of **Cones** and **Rods**. The cones, concentrated where the point of focus normally falls, are adapted for day vision and are particularly sensitive to colour and detail. Distributed concentrically around the cones are the rods which are used for night vision. Night vision depends on the presence of a substance called visual purple (**Rhodopsin**), which takes some 30 min to reach full concentration (**Night Adaptation Time**) but which can be destroyed in a moment by a flash of intense light. Due to the distribution of the rods, it is helpful at night not to look directly at an object, but slightly to one side, so that the rays of light are permitted to fall on the rods and not to be focused on the cones.

The eyes are adapted to terrestrial life where the source of light normally comes from above. They are recessed in cavities and protected from above by the eyebrows and the broad expanse of the overhanging forehead. Each eye is further shielded by two lids. The lower is small and relatively immobile whilst the upper is larger with a wide range of movement. It is the upper lid which moves down to meet the lower lid when the eyes are closed. The amount of light which is allowed to enter the eye depends upon the **Iris**. This circular-shaped and often beautifully pigmented organ of muscular structure surrounds the **Pupil** and functions in a manner similar to the aperture or eye of a camera. By contracting, the size of the pupil is reduced and less light is permitted to enter the eye. By dilating, the pupil increases in size and more light is allowed to enter the eye.

Light, on entering the earth's atmosphere, is scattered by air molecules and particles suspended in the atmosphere. Brightness is an equation between the intensity of the light source and the amount of scatter. Scatter is greater in the denser atmosphere near the earth's surface. Thus, the sky looks progressively darker when viewed with increasing altitude until it resembles our sky at night, as seen from the ground.

2. Reversal of Light Source

When flying at altitude, above cloud, the source of light is reversed, due to the greater intensity of light reflected from the cloud below than the light from the sky above. The instrument panel will be cast into shadow and difficult to read; a situation not made any easier for the pilot by the intense glare entering his eyes from below. The following precautions will help to alleviate this situation—

(*a*) Wear a well fitting pair of anti-glare spectacles.
(*b*) A strong beam of light originating from the cabin roof and focused on the instrument panel is of the greatest help.
(*c*) If you can lower your seat or remove your cushion, then you should do so. This will permit the aircraft to shield you from the glare below.

3. The Empty Visual Field

When flying at altitude or above cloud, if there is no definite pattern of earth or sky for the eye to focus on it will unconsciously take up its position of rest. A speck of dust on the windscreen can, under these circumstances, be mistaken for a distant flying aircraft. A concerted effort to refocus on infinity in order to scan the sky, will be unsuccessful and only result in the eye focusing on a point even nearer to the face.

If there is no definite pattern to be seen in the clouds or on the earth's surface, it is advisable to look out at the wing tip which is the more distant from you. This will cause the eye to change from its position of rest and enable you to focus again on a distant object. This trick must be repeated several times a minute, because the eye will tend to return quickly to its position of rest and fail to refocus on infinity. Having identified an object as an aircraft, it will appear to be further away than it actually is; this is an optical illusion which is seldom fully appreciated. Added to this, it will be impossible to estimate accurately either the aircraft's relative speed or size, since there will be no other object of known size with which to compare it.

An example of this is the sun, which looks much larger when setting than it does when high in the sky. This is because as the sun sets there is a terrestrial reference to the horizon for size comparison, in addition to the refractive properties of the lower atmosphere. Under these circumstances, not only does the sun look larger but it appears to change colour and to assume the appearance of a red ball. This is explained by the fact that those colours with a shorter wavelength are absorbed by the thick dust in the earth's lower atmosphere, and only the reds, which occupy the other end of the visual spectrum, can penetrate this particle barrier.

4. Visual Illusions at Night

(a) AUTO-KINETIC ILLUSION

A point source of light when viewed against a featureless dark background will appear to oscillate when, in fact, it is motionless; a state of affairs which is known as the **Auto-kinetic Illusion**. The degree of apparent movement will increase if the object is allowed to become the prime focus of attention. To lessen the effects of this visual illusion it is necessary only to shift the gaze in order not to stare with fixed concentration at such a source of light.

(b) OCULOGYRAL ILLUSION

Another visual illusion commonly encountered in night flying is known as the **Oculogyral Illusion**. If a source of light is viewed from an aircraft which itself is the subject of considerable angular acceleration, the light source will appear to develop a movement of its own and this apparent movement may continue for some time after straight and level flight has been resumed. This illusion is produced by involuntary eye movements (**Nystagmus**) which are caused by vestibular inspired impulses reaching the brain from the semicircular canals. Vestibular function is discussed in Chapter 4 but it is convenient at this point to emphasize that the frequency and amplitude of these involuntary eye movements, and therefore the character of the illusion itself, will vary directly with the forces created by angular acceleration. It is for this reason that, whilst flying at night, care should be taken not to initiate manoeuvres which could create considerable angular acceleration forces.

(c) THE UPSIDE-DOWN ILLUSION

This illusion could affect the private pilot soaring to very high altitudes in mountain-wave formation at night. Due to the considerable height and the curvature of the earth's surface both the nose and wing tips will appear to be well above the horizon and there will be a very noticeable amount of sky below the aircraft. Under these conditions, if the moon is seen below the aircraft but above the horizon and there is no clear pattern of stars above the aircraft, conflict and confusion can be caused which may result in the pilot becoming convinced that he is flying upside down.

5. Visual Standards

Amblyopia, or inadequate vision due to errors of refraction, lack of ocular muscle balance or defective colour perception, is responsible for many people, who are otherwise healthy, failing to reach the medical standards required for the issue or renewal of a Flying Licence. This chapter has been written in a sincere attempt to explain in simple language the Romano-Greek terminology of the Ophthalmologist or Eye Specialist.

6. Visual Acuity

This means the ability to see, and is assessed by confronting the candidate with one of Snellen's Test Type Cards suitably illuminated and placed at a distance of 6 metres. This test is based on the assumption that the average normal eye is able to see clearly a letter whose overall size subtends an angle of 5 min of arc as it reaches the eye and the width of each stroke of each letter subtends an angle of 1 min of arc at the eye. Since the standard testing distance is 6 m, it follows that all vision is recorded in the 6-m notation; the numerator, or figure above the line in the fraction, indicating the test distance and the denominator, or figure below the line in the fraction, indicating the distance at which the test letter should be clearly see. Thus the fraction 6/6 means that at a distance of 6 m the eye can read those letters which are intended to be read by the normal eye at a distance of 6 metres. The fraction 6/9 means that the eye at a distance of 6 m can only read those (larger) letters intended to be read by the normal eye at a distance of 9 m.

7. Visual Acuity of the Student/Private Pilot

This should be at least 6/12 in each eye separately, with or without correcting glasses. The vision without glasses in either or both eyes must not be less than 6/60. Under these conditions, the candidate may be assessed fit for a licence, subject to the requirements that approved glasses are worn whilst exercising the privileges of this type of Flying Licence.

8. Visual Acuity of the Airline Transport and Commercial Pilot

This is of a higher standard than that of a student or private pilot and must be at least 6/9 in each eye separately, with or without glasses. If this visual acuity is obtained only by the use of correcting glasses in either or both eyes, it must not be less than 6/18 without glasses. In this case the candidate may be assessed fit for a licence, subject to the requirement that approved glasses are worn whilst exercising the privileges of this type of Flying Licence.

9. Emmetropia

This is the healthy state where, when the eye is fully relaxed, parallel rays of light are focused on the retina.

10. Hypermetropia

This is that state where, when the eye is fully relaxed, parallel rays of light are focused behind the retina, either because the eyeball axis is too short or because the refractive power of the eye is too weak. This refractive error can be overcome to a greater or lesser extent by a conscious effort which will result in clearer vision. Hypermetropic refractive errors are treated with convex lenses.

11. Manifest Hypermetropia

This is a measure of the refractive error which can be overcome by the candidate with hypermetropia and may be given by the power of the strongest convex lens through which the

6/6 line can be read. Since the power of a lens is expressed in dioptres, the degree of **Manifest Hypermetropia** is stated numerically in dioptres. A reading of more than $+2\cdot25$ dioptres at the initial examination for a Commercial or Airline Transport Pilot's Licence would be regarded as unacceptable.

12. Presbyopia

This is that state of long-sightedness which afflicts an individual later in life and is usually noticed for the first time in the early forties. It is not difficult to spot the presbyopic person for he or she can be seen peering and squinting in obvious difficulty when confronted with the small print of a standard telephone directory. Their difficulty arises from age changes within the substance of the lens of the eye which makes it less pliable and less able to accommodate in order to focus on a near object. These individuals, as a rule, have good distance vision but need the help of glasses for reading or close work. Presbyopic pilots can be seen peering through their half-glasses when reading their maps but happily looking over the top of their spectacles when scanning the sky for other aircraft.

13. Myopia

This is that state where, when the eye is fully relaxed, parallel rays of light are focused in front of the retina either because the eyeball axis is too long or the refractive power of the eye is too strong. The condition is treated with concave lenses which must be worn at all times for distance vision, for these people are short-sighted.

14. Astigmatism

This relates to abnormalities of the curvature of the surface of the cornea, and to a much smaller extent, the surface of the lens. In simple terms, the healthy cornea is spheroidal shaped, like a "soccer" ball, whilst the astigmatic cornea is oval shaped, like a "rugger" ball. The errors of refraction caused by an astigmatic cornea are correctable by cylindrical lenses.

15. Anisometropia

This term describes a difference in the refractive index of each eye and can be associated with problems which involve diplopia, or double vision.

16. Accommodation

Accommodation, or near vision, may be measured both uni-ocularly and binocularly, with an instrument called the R.A.F. Near Point Rule. The ability to accommodate or adjust for near vision decreases with age, due to changes within the lens which make it less pliable and reduce its ability to refract.

17. Convergence

This is the ability to follow an object with both eyes as it draws closer and to see it clearly. This single object when viewed binocularly as it approaches, will first become blurred and then later become double. This test may also be carried out with the R.A.F. Near Point Rule and the point of subjective convergence (sensed by the subject and not observed by the examiner) is reached when the object becomes double, and this distance is measured in centimetres.

18. Ocular Muscle Balance

This depends on the action of the extrinsic and intrinsic muscles of the eye being co-ordinated by a complex neuro-muscular mechanism which results in the visual axes of both eyes being directed towards any object which at the time is the focus of attention. In this state of **Orthophoria,** if binocular vision is interrupted, both visual axes should remain directed towards the object. Heterophoria is that condition of the eyes in which the visual axes fail to maintain their normal direction when the stimulus of binocular vision is temporarily removed, resulting in convergence (**Esophoria**), divergence (**Exophoria**) or vertical deviation either upwards or downwards (**Hyperphoria** or **Hypophoria**). These states constitute the various forms of latent squint or **Strabismus** and are important for they may give rise to blurring of vision, headaches or double vision, especially when a pilot is tired after a prolonged period of instrument flying and may lead to accidents by a failure to estimate height correctly when on the approach and landing.

19. Colour Perception

Defective colour perception is a permanent condition present at birth. Colour vision is tested when the student pilot presents himself for his initial medical examination. On this occasion, he will be confronted with a set of colour charts (Ishihara Test). If his answers are correct he will be regarded as having normal colour perception. However, should he fail, he will be subjected to a lantern test (The Giles Archer Aviation Lantern is used for this test). Depending on the result of this test, he will be graded as either **Colour Defective Safe** or **Colour Defective Unsafe,** depending on whether or not he can distinguish accurately between red, green and white lights.

4. The Ear and Hearing

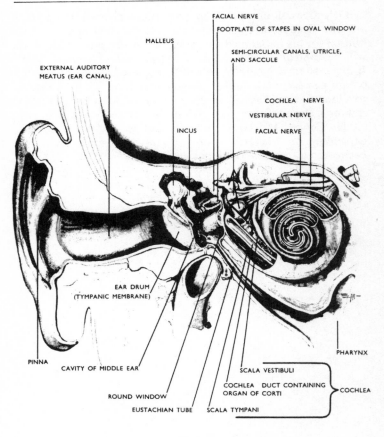

FACIAL NERVE

FOOTPLATE OF STAPES IN OVAL WINDOW

MALLEUS

SEMI-CIRCULAR CANALS, UTRICLE, AND SACCULE

EXTERNAL AUDITORY MEATUS (EAR CANAL)

COCHLEA NERVE

VESTIBULAR NERVE

INCUS

FACIAL NERVE

EAR DRUM (TYMPANIC MEMBRANE)

PHARYNX

PINNA

CAVITY OF MIDDLE EAR

SCALA VESTIBULI

COCHLEA DUCT CONTAINING ORGAN OF CORTI

COCHLEA

ROUND WINDOW

EUSTACHIAN TUBE

SCALA TYMPANI

FIG. 3. The Human Ear

40

1. The Ear

The human ear has two functions—

(*a*) The sense of hearing.
(*b*) The sense of balance.

For descriptive purposes the ear is divided into three parts; the **Outer,** the **Middle,** and the **Inner Ear.** The inner ear contains the labyrinthine apparatus which is divided into two parts according to function—

(*a*) The **Cochlea,** which includes the organ of corti, is responsible for hearing.
(*b*) The non-acoustic or **Vestibular** apparatus, which is responsible for balance.

2. Sense of Hearing

Sound waves, which are directed down the **External Auditory Canal,** cause the **Ear Drum** or **Tympanic Membrane** to vibrate. These vibrations are amplified and conducted across the middle ear by three small bones (**Malleus, Incus, Stapes**) to the **Inner Ear** where the **Cochlea,** which is the organ of hearing, converts them to nerve impulses which are relayed to the brain by the cochlea nerve.

The **middle ear** is an air-filled cavity within the bony skull and is connected to the **Naso-Pharynx,** that space behind the nose, by the **Eustachian Tube.** This tube provides the means by which a two-way flow of air can enter and leave the middle ear and facilitates the equalization of air pressure on both sides of the ear drum.

In sustained climbs the ambient air pressure will fall and unless air can escape, a relatively high-pressure system will develop in the middle ear and cause the ear drum to bulge outwards. For air to escape from the middle ear through the Eustachian tubes a head of pressure is required. As this air "vents off" the pilot will become aware of his ears "popping" and clearing in sequential step-ladder heights of approximately 350 ft. Conversely, when descending, a low-pressure system will develop in the middle ear and the ear drum will tend to bulge inwards. Because the mucous membrane, which lines the Eustachian tubes, is set in folds and acts like a non-return valve, it is more difficult for air to enter the middle ear than to leave it. Therefore it is not uncommon for healthy people to experience some discomfort in the ears during descent and under these circumstances it is often helpful to swallow repeatedly. Each act of swallowing will, by the muscular movements involved, help to part the folds within the Eustachian Tubes and encourage the passage of air to the middle ears. If the ears should remain blocked regardless of the efforts being made to clear them a potentially serious situation will arise and very great care should be taken to prevent rupture of one or both ear drums. The rate of descent should be decreased, or even some altitude regained, and the patient advised to take deep breaths and blow hard whilst pinching the nose and pursing the lips; sniffing naso-pharyngeal decongestants may also help to clear the Eustachian Tubes. "Blocked ears" are associated with the **Common Cold, Sinusitis, Tonsilitis,** or indeed any infection or allergic condition capable of causing catarrh or swelling of the tissues in and around the Eustachian Tubes.

Rupture of the ear drum (**Otitic Barotrauma**) is preceded by pain so intense that the pilot may be unable to maintain control over his aircraft or be able to fly safely even under the most favourable conditions. Ear-drum rupture is a serious condition which should receive expert medical attention if permanent injury is to be avoided. Untreated, it is not likely that the hole will heal spontaneously and subsequent scar tissue formation could cause a conductive type of deafness. Unless protected by an intact ear drum, the middle ear may become the site of re-peated attacks of infection which could cause a foul smelling discharge from the ear and give rise to sudden disabling attacks of giddiness. If in doubt as to whether you will be able to clear your ears in the air, carry out a simple check on the ground by pinching the nostrils and blowing with the mouth closed; when you do this both ears should pop. Finally, do not hesitate to ground yourself if you think your ears are blocked, for it is much wiser to seek medical advice than to risk serious and unpleasant complications at a later date. It is, of course, possible that you will be found to be suffering from an accumulation of wax in the ears; a condition quickly relieved by gentle syringeing.

SINUS BAROTRAUMA

The **Paranasal Sinuses** are cavities within the bones which constitute part of the face and skull. They are connected to the **Nasal Cavity** by narrow ducts which, like the sinuses themselves, are lined by mucous membrane particularly sensitive to the sense of smell. The size and shape of these cavities affects the tone of the human voice. In the healthy state, air flows freely through the nasal and paranasal cavities and maintains equality with the ambient cabin air pressure. Trouble arises and can become serious if this free flow of air is interrupted by partial or complete blockage of the paranasal ducts. This state of affairs may arise from a variety of causes and those most commonly encountered in aviation are the common cold (**Acute Coryza**) and hay fever (**Allergic Rhinitis**). Pressure differences of this nature, which will be experienced both during ascent and descent, may cause pain so severe as to render a pilot quite incapable of maintaining control of his aircraft. This condition which is known as **Sinus Barotrauma** may be accompanied by watering of the eyes, headache and pain affecting both cheeks and forehead. This condition, like otitic barotrauma, is serious and is a valid reason for temporary grounding until treatment has proved effective. Sinus barotrauma is most likely to occur at heights below 20000 ft.

3. Noise

Acoustically, sound vibrations or pressure waves contain two variable factors.

- (*a*) The **Intensity of Sound** will depend on the amplitude of the sound waves and will be registered as **Loudness.**
- (*b*) The **Frequency** or cycles per second (c/s or Hz) of the sound waves will be registered as **Pitch.**

The smallest force capable of causing the normal ear drum to vibrate sufficiently to penetrate the **Threshold of Hearing** is a pressure change at the ear drum of 0·0002 dynes per sq. cm. at 1000 c/s. Units of sound are measured in decibels (dB) and one such unit represents the lowest change in sound level which the healthy youthful ear can detect. For any given sound, the intensity in dB is—

$$20 \log_{10} \frac{\text{(Pressure on the external surface of the ear drum in dynes per sq. cm.)}}{0·0002}$$

The audible effect of sound intensities may be illustrated by the following examples—

0 dB	Threshold of hearing.
15 dB	Whisper.
30 dB	Conversation at home.
45 dB	Conversation in busy office.
60 dB	Noise level in a crowded street.
80 dB	Full orchestra playing a loud passage of music.
120 dB	Piston engine noise, a few feet away.
130 dB	Jet aircraft noise, a few feet away.
150 dB	Jet aircraft with after-burner selected.

The **Frequency Range** of human hearing extends from 20 c/s to 15 000 c/s and may be illustrated by the following examples—

50–100 c/s	The hum originating from "mains voltage" electrical equipment working on 50 c/s.
256 c/s	Middle "C" on the piano.
300–5000 c/s	Speech intelligibility range.
8000 c/s	Represents upper level of speech frequencies.

SOME EFFECTS OF NOISE LEVELS

1. 120 dB will cause discomfort in the ears.
2. 140 dB will cause pain in the ears.
3. Sustained noise levels above 85 dB can lead to temporary or permanent hearing loss.

4. Exposure to levels above 120 dB for several hours a day for 3 to 6 months will cause deafness.
5. Noises of 100 dB in the frequency range below 100 c/s will cause the body to vibrate whilst noises in excess of 150 dB will cause sweating to occur between the fingers and under the collar.
6. High intensity noises can affect co-ordination of mental and physical activity and lead to disorientation.
7. High intensity noises, below the dangerous level, must be regarded as stress factors capable of leading to an overall reduction in efficiency.

Slightly more than one per cent of the total power output of a jet engine is in the form of noise, the frequency of which will extend over the entire range of audibility and also give rise to ultrasonic oscillations. In the open air, noise dispersal will obey the inverse square law and diminish by 6 dB as the distance from the sound is doubled. In confined spaces, this law is not applicable, for sounds will be reflected and may even be intensified. Some concern is being felt in this respect by operators of helicopters powered by gas-turbine engines for in these aircraft the compressors are often in very close proximity to the crew. Individuals who are constantly exposed to jet-engine noise are at risk and special precautions should be taken to prevent the onset of high-tone deafness. In the early stages of this type of deafness the individual may be unaware of his incapacity, for it will be limited to the upper frequency noises (above 4000 c/s), but in time, however, loss of auditory acuity will extend into the normal speech frequencies and the individual will then become conscious of the fact that he is going deaf.

PROTECTION AGAINST NOISE.

Well fitting ear plugs will provide attenuation protection of the order of 25 dB, whilst ear muffs will provide protection of the order of 45 dB at the higher frequencies.

Noise conducted through the bone structure of the skull and face is about 40 dB below that conducted through air conduction via the ear drum and middle ear. Thus, however efficient ear protection may be it can never give more than 40 dB protection. It is therefore important that individuals who are concerned in the operation of jet aircraft should wear, in addition to ear protectors, a well fitting helmet or bone dome.

TOXIC DEAFNESS

This condition may be caused by alcoholism or heavy smoking. Deafness associated with "Ringing" or **Tinnitus** in the ears may result from taking such drugs as Aspirin, Quinine, Sulphonamides and Streptomycin.

PRESBYACUSIS

This is the name given to the condition of deteriorating auditory acuity associated with growing old. The normal loss in hearing ability which can be expected by the sixth decade is of the order of 5 per cent and by the seventh decade 10 per cent.

4. The Sense of Balance

Man, a relatively slow-moving land creature, is remarkably well adapted to contend with the conditions of his normal terrestrial environment. Even in the absence of visual reference, a blind man can maintain effective balance over a wide range of movements whilst walking over uneven ground simply by automatic reaction to reliable sensations which reach his brain from the vestibular apparatus and sensors in the muscles, joints and skin. It is when man leaves his normal environment to take to the air that he finds himself, for the first time, ill-adapted and inadequately equipped by evolutionary development to interpret and react correctly to acceleration forces of infinitely greater magnitude and duration than those he is accustomed to experience on the ground. It is under these circumstances, when unaided by visual reference to the horizon, that he may be so overwhelmed by misleading and contradictory bodily sensations that he may lose all sense of spatial orientation and cease to have any knowledge of his bodily attitude in relationship to the earth's surface.

It is this state which is implied by the term **Disorientation.** Thus, on the ground man is able to maintain balance without visual reference but in the air his ability to orientate himself will depend on visual reference alone. Under visual meteorological conditions, orientation is maintained by reference to the earth's horizon, but under instrument meteorological conditions the pilot must learn to interpret visually attitude information displayed on the instrument panel and have the ability to disbelieve, or the will power to ignore, all other bodily sensations.

It is this requirement that man finds so difficult to learn and once learned can so easily forget if he does not keep himself in constant practice. It is for these reasons that whilst flying on instruments the pilot's attention must be directed to a repeated sequence of actions which will include checking the power setting, checking the attitude, checking the trim and then checking the other instruments until free of cloud and in clear visual reference with the ground.

5. The Vestibular Apparatus

The Vestibular Apparatus consists of the **Semicircular Canals** and **Otolith Organ** which is divided into two parts called respectively the **Utricle** and **Saccule.**

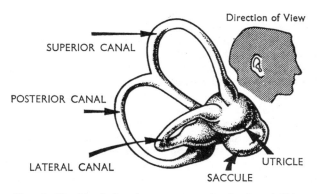

Fig. 4. The Vestibular Apparatus on the Starboard Side

6. The Function of the Semicircular Canals

In each ear there are three fluid-filled semicircular canals which are set in three planes at right-angles to one another. At the base of each canal is a sensory organ called the **Cupula** which is a flap-like valve, anchored at one end and consisting of hair-like nerve endings enclosed within a capsule. During rotational movements of the head, the fluid within the canal, due to inertia, lags behind and deflects the cupula. When the fluid has overcome its inertia, the cupula will return once more to its position of rest and cease to send any messages to the brain via the vestibular nerve.

When rotation in this plane stops, the fluid within the canals, again because of inertia, will cause a deflection of the cupula, but this time in the opposite direction. Since there are three canals set at right angles to one another, forces due to acceleration can be registered in yaw, pitch and roll simultaneously. Thus, in the absence of visual cues, the brain will interpret stimuli arising from the semicircular canals in the following manner—

(*a*) Acceleration as movement.

(*b*) Changing rates of acceleration for acceleration itself.

(*c*) Constant velocity as rest.

7. The Function of the Otolith Organ

This organ is sensitive to the direction and force of gravity. In changing positions of the head it is sensitive to the magnitude and direction of the apparent gravitational pull. This apparent pull is the resultant force of the earth's actual gravitational pull and the forces due to acceleration. It is similar therefore to the ball in a turn-and-slip indicator, where the ball indicates the degree of balance of the turn. When an aircraft is slipping into the centre of a turn, the ball will be deflected towards the lower wing and more rudder, applied in the direction of the lower wing, will be required to balance the turn and centralize the ball. When an aircraft is skidding out of a turn, the ball will be deflected towards the upper wing and less rudder will be required to balance the turn and centralize the ball.

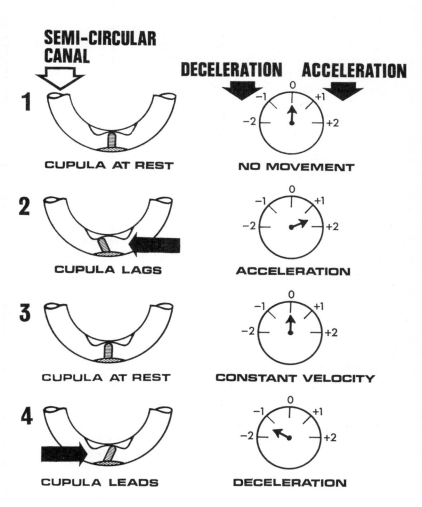

FIG. 5. Cupula Response to Acceleration

8. Vestibular Response to a Rate One Turn

A simple example of the effect of vestibular dynamics may be experienced during prolonged rotational movements which accompany a **Rate One Turn.** On entering such a turn, forces due to angular acceleration will cause cupula deflection by fluid flow inertia within the semicircular canals. Once the turn has been established, and has been maintained for some twenty seconds, the effects of inertia will have been overcome and cupula deflection will have ceased. Thus, even though the body may be experiencing considerable angular velocity, there will be no conscious appreciation of rotation from this vestibular source. When the turn is stopped in order to resume straight-and-level flight, rotational forces will cease abruptly and the resultant fluid surge within the semicircular canals will cause cupula deflection in the opposite direction. This change in flow will register a rate of turn which is both equal and opposite to that which has been occurring, but which in fact has just ceased. These sensations will persist until inertia has once again been overcome and cupula deflection has stopped. Thus, during these gentle manoeuvres the pilot has received two very misleading vestibular messages. Firstly, there was no sensation of turning whilst a turn was actually taking place, and secondly there was a feeling of turning at a time when no such turn was taking place and, in fact, when straight-and-level flight had been resumed.

9. Vestibular Response to Spinning and Spin Recovery

Misleading vestibular sensations are further exaggerated when forces due to angular acceleration are of increased magnitude and are occurring in more than one plane at the same time. For example, nodding movements of the head occurring whilst other rotational movements are taking place in a different plane can give rise to considerable mental confusion and lead to disorientation. Relatively large forces, due to acceleration, are imposed on the semicircular canals by relatively small angular movements of the head because the radius of rotation of the head is so short. The after-effects of spin recovery will be less disturbing if, during the spinning phase, the eyes are allowed to follow the horizon rather than being fixed on a point on the the ground. To understand this fully, it must be realized that if the eyes are directed onto the ground during the spin the after-sensation will be one of rotation about an axis, from front to back, through the head. When recovery action has proved effective and the aircraft is being eased out of the subsequent dive, backward rotation of the head will be necessary if the eyes are to be allowed to meet the horizon as it enters the visual field from above. Rotation of the head in this plane, which will be at right-angles to the after-sensation of spinning, can prove very disturbing but if, during the act of spinning and subsequent spin recovery, the head is held still and the eyes are directed at the horizon all the time, no such movement of the head will be necessary and far less confusion will follow. Finally, it may be added that a downward glance with the eyes, without moving the head, will prove sufficient to scan the instruments during these manoeuvres.

10. Vestibular Response to Rapid Linear Acceleration

It will be seen in Fig. 6A that a pilot, when flying at constant speed, will experience a vertical force due to gravity, represented by line *ab*, and will interpret this as weight.

If, at this stage, the pilot should decide to increase the aircraft's speed, in straight-and-level flight, by increasing thrust he will experience an additional force, due to bodily inertia, represented by the line *ac* in Fig. 6B. During this phase of linear acceleration, the pilot's vestibular apparatus (in this case mostly of otolith origin) will resolve these forces into an apparent vertical resultant force, represented by the line *ad*, which will give a bodily sensation which will make the unwary pilot think that his aircraft has adopted a nose-up attitude in pitch. Thus, again, in the absence of visual reference, the pilot must believe what his instruments tell him and ignore his false bodily sensations.

11. Vestibular Response to Rapid Linear Deceleration

It will be seen from Fig. 6C that during deceleration, in straight-and-level flight, the apparent vertical resultant force

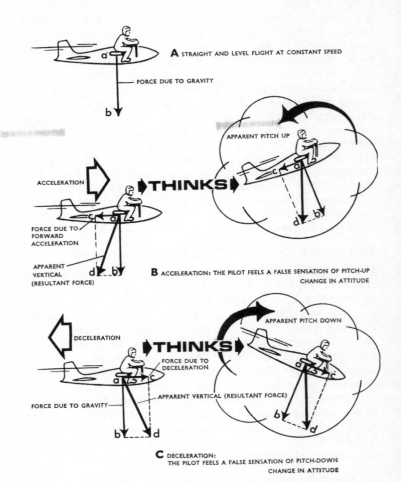

FIG. 6. Representation of False Sensations arising from Acceleration and Deceleration

will make the unwary pilot feel that his aircraft has adopted a nose-down attitude in pitch. Once again, he must believe his instruments and ignore his bodily sensations if he is to fly accurately and safely.

12. Vestibular Response to Sudden Linear Acceleration and Deceleration

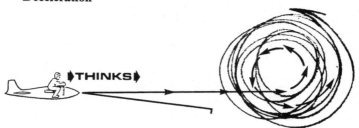

FIG. 7A. Sudden Linear Acceleration—Catapult, Snatch or Rocket 'Launch'

These forces will produce the sensation of rotating backwards, heels over head

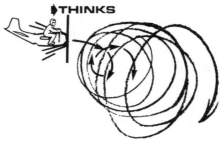

FIG. 7B. Sudden Linear Deceleration—Crash Impact, Arrester Wires or Crash Barrier

These forces will produce the sensation of rotating forwards, head over heels

Figs. 7A and 7B show how, under conditions of sudden acceleration and deceleration, the vestibular apparatus produces the most alarming and false sensations which even the pilot's visual reference will not be strong enough to overcome.

13. Forces Due to Acceleration

Forces due to acceleration are usually measured in units of earth's gravity. One "g" is the force required to accelerate a body at 32·2 ft per sec. per sec. The human body is not affected by speed but is greatly affected by forces due to acceleration which may themselves vary in magnitude, direction and duration. In forced landings and ditchings linear deceleration forces may exceed 10 "g" and it has been shown that, properly supported, the human body can withstand forces far in excess of an aircraft structure. In general terms, it is not necessary to provide protection against linear deceleration forces greater than 25 "g", since values of this order will be associated with disintegration of the aircraft itself. During violent deceleration the occupant may be flung forwards and injured or killed by striking objects in front of the seat. Where provided, the conventional seat harness, combining a lap belt and shoulder restraints, must be worn at all times by the pilot and passengers of light aircraft and gliders. During pre-flight checks particular attention should be paid to ensure that the lap belt is fitting tightly and is positioned as low as possible and that the shoulder straps are tight and locked. A high-fitting lap belt will allow the wearer to slip under the harness during linear deceleration forces. Accident investigations have focused attention on the strength of the holding points of the seat harnesses, particularly in gliders. It is possible that fatal injuries have resulted, not from a failure of the harnesses themselves, but from a collapse of their anchor points on the glider.

Forces due to deceleration during parachute deployment may, for a 24-ft canopy, exceed 30 "g" at 32000 ft and could cause disintegration of the parachute material. At heights below 10000 ft the shock load is approximately 8 "g".

14. Positive and Negative "g".

Positive "g" is produced when centrifugal force, created by angular acceleration, is applied to a pilot and acts from his head to his feet.

Negative "g" is produced when centrifugal force, created by angular acceleration, is applied to a pilot and acts from his feet to his head.

Positive "g" is therefore experienced when doing a turn or inside loop and negative "g" when doing an outside loop or bunt.

The force produced by such manoeuvres is given by the formula—

$$F = \frac{MV^2}{R}$$

where F = The force produced by acceleration.

M = Mass of aircraft.

R = Radius of turn.

V = Velocity.

From this formula it will be seen that—

(a) If the velocity is doubled, the force is quadrupled.

(b) If the radius of the turn is halved, the force is doubled.

These forces are felt by the pilot as an increase or decrease in weight. Weight varies directly with acceleration because

weight = mass × acceleration, mass remaining constant.

15. The Effects of Increased Positive "g" on the Pilot

The skin, underlying connective tissue and muscles will be forced downwards towards the lower extremities. The pilot will become aware that his face is elongating, his jaw is being drawn down and his mouth is being forced open. His arms and legs will feel heavy and he will be unable to rise from the sitting position when experiencing forces in excess of 2·5 positive "g". The heart, which is a strong muscular pump responsible for circulating the blood around the body, is normally situated in the centre of the chest behind the breast bone. The apex of the heart may be felt beating on the left side of the chest in the space between the fifth and sixth ribs, about 3·5 in. from the midline.

Under increased positive "g" the heart is displaced downwards and the arteries connecting it to the brain will be stretched and elongated. The blood contained within these blood vessels will weigh more because of the increased "g". Thus, blood flow to all parts of the body above the heart, including the upper and middle lobes of the lungs, will be reduced whilst those parts of the body below the heart will become increasingly engorged with blood. Blood will tend to pool in the vascular spaces in the lower abdomen and legs and diminish the venous return to the heart and therefore reduce the circulating blood volume. All these factors combine to diminish the supply of well oxygenated blood to the brain, which, like all nervous tissue, is particularly sensitive to hypoxia.

Individual reaction to positive "g" varies and short, thin pilots have an advantage over their more generously built colleagues, but the following is a reasonable guide to the effects—

(a) Partial loss of vision, which is called **Greying out,** will occur if between 3 and 4 "g" is applied for 5 sec.

(b) Total loss of vision, which is called **Blacking Out**, will occur if 5 "g" is applied for 5 sec. and may be followed by unconsciousness.

Because a passenger will tend to black out before the pilot, the latter is not justified in thinking that he is made of sterner stuff. The probable explanation lies in the fact that the pilot knows what is about to happen and braces himself subconsciously by tensing the leg and abdominal muscles in an effort to reduce the amount of pooling of blood in the lower extremities.

Positive "g" loadings in excess of those required to produce blacking out will cause increasing degrees of hypoxia of the brain and give rise to mental confusion and unconsciousness. Once the "g" forces are removed recovery begins immediately but 30 sec. or more may elapse before full clarity of mind is restored.

16. The Effects of Negative "g" on the Pilot

A force of one negative "g" is experienced during inverted straight-and-level flight. Any increase of negative "g" applied

when performing an outside loop or bunt produces effects both
unpleasant and possibly dangerous. Blood is forced into the head
and neck, and the soft tissues including the lower eyelids become
engorged. The applied centrifugal force causes the lower eyelids
to cover the pupils as they move towards the retreating upper
eyelids. Light will then enter the eye through the tissues of the
lower eyelid and the subject will become conscious of a misty
redness. This sequence is responsible for the term **"Red-Out"**.
The small unsupported blood vessels under the conjunctiva
covering the whites of the eyes may rupture and give rise to sub-
conjunctival haemorrhages which, while not affecting vision,
will prove unsightly and may take six to ten days to clear.
Tolerance to negative "g" is less than to positive "g" and prolonged negative "g" will give rise to symptoms similar to those
of concussion. Aerobatics involving extremes of these forces are
better avoided.

17. Disorientation

The human eye is the supreme soloist in the sensory orchestra
and, whilst other sensors may play their many parts, the eye
remains the supreme master of **Spatial Orientation.** Alone it is
capable of creating order out of chaos and of resolving the
problems of disorientation, for in the absence of visual reference
to the true horizon it can be used to interpret information displayed on the instrument panel. It is no mystery why birds do
not fly in cloud; it is because nature has not provided them with
an artificial horizon.

In conditions of clear visibility little difficulty is experienced
in ignoring misleading vestibular messages, since a reassuring
glance at the horizon will bring comfort and a return of confi-
dence to a mind which has begun to suffer from the twin
emotions of conflict and confusion . . . a state of affairs implied by the term disorientation.

When in cloud or at night, the experienced pilot in current
practice will have no difficulty in flying on instruments, for he
has learned to disregard all information except visual appreciation of his instruments. It is under conditions of haze and poor

visibility in broken cloud, when the pilot's attention is employed searching for a ground reference, that trouble is likely to arise. It is in those brief moments when the pilot's eyes are distracted from his instruments that misleading bodily sensations may cause the unwary pilot to make inappropriate control movements and allow the aircraft to get into an attitude from which it is difficult to recover on instruments alone. A glider pilot entering a thunder cloud may experience extreme turbulence and, more often, when he is learning, the unfortunate fellow will find himself the victim of one of nature's most powerful displays of force. The turbulence may be so violent that his aircraft could be thrown into attitudes far beyond the limits of an artificial horizon, and, without visual cues, he may find himself the recipient of conflicting and totally misleading vestibular messages. In his panic he may execute wild attempts at recovery action, but since he is now disorientated, his efforts are only likely to make matters worse. These control movements may subject him to rapidly changing and ever-increasing forces due to acceleration and bring about a series of blackouts, complicated by a state of near collapse, giddiness, and motion sickness. Add to this scene those conditions which exist within a thunder cloud, namely, rain, hailstones, snow, thunder, lightning, St. Elmo's Fire, electric shocks, and the noise of ice cracking and breaking away from the surface of the aircraft, and you will have a vivid picture of the horror and dangers associated with the state of disorientation. In the happy event of the aircraft surviving these conditions, and presuming he is still conscious, it will take the pilot a further thirty seconds or more, after being spewed out of cloud, to recover sufficiently to orientate himself by visual reference to the ground.

If forced to bale out in a thunder cloud, it is probably wiser not to use your parachute until you have fallen free of cloud. By deploying a parachute in the middle of a thunder cloud, it is possible to be carried upwards, in rapidly rising air at speeds in excess of fifty feet a second, to altitudes where hypoxia can render a pilot unconscious and exposure can freeze him to death.

18. Vertigo and Motion Sickness

The term **Vertigo** is used to indicate disorientation which may include a sensation of giddiness and is usually caused by rapidly changing forces due to linear, radial, and angular acceleration. It may also be caused by disordered function of the vestibular apparatus, due to disease, or may happen quite suddenly when blowing the nose or sneezing violently. In either case, an explosive change of air pressure in the naso-pharynx is transmitted via the Eustachian Tube to the middle ear where, via the round window, it so disturbs the vestibular apparatus in the adjoining inner ear that a violent barrage of conflicting vestibular messages is fed to the brain.

Motion Sickness is a clinical manifestation of vestibular excitation, for it is known that individuals without a functioning vestibular apparatus do not suffer from this condition. **Air Sickness,** like car sickness or sea sickness, is a relatively common condition which affects children and adults who are said to be of a nervous disposition. This apprehension, if it exists, is really the fear of the thought of being sick and this fact alone goes a long way to explain why individuals of the stomach and courage of Nelson can be incapacitated by motion sickness.

Drugs recommended for the relief of motion sickness should be taken only on medical advice and should never be prescribed for the lone aviator, because motion sickness drugs produce cerebral sedation as well as reducing vestibular response to rotational movements. The treatment of motion sickness is discussed in Chapter 5.

5. Diseases, Drugs and Drink

1. Am I Fit to Fly?

Many otherwise avoidable flying accidents have resulted from one, or a combination of the following three: **diseases, drugs,** and **drink.** Many illnesses, which on the ground are of trivial inconvenience, can assume dangerous proportions in the air and cause fatal crashes. Diseases which may cause physical symptoms can also be associated with disturbing mental complications, for it is known that marked deterioration in flying skill can result from the common cold, sinusitis, minor chest infections, lumbago or even a full bladder. As new and more powerful drugs are introduced, more and more side effects are becoming apparent. If you feel unwell your symptoms may be the result of your illness, or of the drugs which you have taken to combat it. You must therefore ask yourself the following questions—

(a) Am I physically fit to fly an aircraft?

(b) Do I need to continue to take the medicines that have been prescribed for me?

(c) Have the drugs which I have been taking, since I became ill, adversely affected my ability to fly safely?

(d) Am I worried or emotionally upset; if so, should I fly?

If you still remain in doubt about your ability to fly safely after having asked yourself these questions, then you should consult a physician skilled in aviation medicine—or, in the U.K., telephone the Medical Branch, The Board of Trade, Shell Mex House, London.

2. Diseases Which Can Cause Mental Confusion and Unconsciousness

These diseases, such as **Epilepsy, Diabetes and High Blood Pressure,** can render a passenger an unwelcome guest aboard a light aircraft or glider. Such people have been the cause of fatal accidents.

3. Hypoglycaemia

This is a condition in which the sugar content of the blood has fallen to dangerously low levels (in the region of 50 mg per 100 ml of blood) and is associated with the onset of lassitude and drowsiness or light-headedness, leading to a state of collapse and unconsciousness. It can occur as a result of disease (tumours of the pancreas) or result from an overdose of Insulin in an otherwise well controlled diabetic. It may, however, occur in the healthy individual who has been without food for many hours and is suddenly subjected to physical exercise or mental anxiety. For the Private Pilot, it is only necessary to emphasize that it is never wise to fly on an empty stomach and, if a long cross-country flight is planned, a few glucose-containing sweets should be consumed or tea or coffee containing sugar should be drunk during the flight.

4. Carbon Monoxide Poisoning

Carbon monoxide poisoning has been responsible for fatal flying accidents. One of the products of combustion in the petrol engine, it is present in the exhaust gases, which are often harnessed to produce cabin heat by being ducted through a heat exchanger in the aircraft. Even a small leak of this noxious gas into the interior of the aircraft may prove most dangerous for it has an affinity 200 times greater than oxygen for haemoglobin, with which it combines to form **Carboxyhaemoglobin.** Thus, not only is the amount of circulating oxygen reduced, but a side effect of carbon monoxide actively impedes the release of oxygen to the tissues. The effects of carbon monoxide poisoning tend to be insidious, for the gas is odourless and the symptoms it produces are similar to those of hypoxia, but in this case the victim will have a cherry-red colour and the symptoms can occur at altitudes far lower than if due to hypoxia alone. The immediate treatment is twofold: the alleviation of shock, and the displacement of carbon monoxide from the blood and its replacement by oxygen.

Thus the patient needs as much fresh air as possible and oxygen whenever available. The effect of treatment in a hyperbaric chamber, where oxygen can be provided at a pressure of two atmospheres is absolutely dramatic. Under these conditions the affinity of carbon monoxide for haemoglobin is completely overwhelmed and it is rapidly replaced by oxygen. A deeply unconscious patient will recover consciousness in a matter of minutes, whereas ordinary methods of resuscitation may take several hours.

5. Aspirin

Aspirin and compound tablets containing aspirin together with Phenacetin, Codeine or Caffeine are probably the most frequently consumed drugs which can be purchased over the counter and are used effectively to relieve many minor ailments. If taken in normal dosage, the side effects are not likely to prove embarrassing, but in larger doses gastric irritation may cause bleeding to occur from the lining of the stomach. Vomiting of blood, due to this cause, can be associated with sudden collapse; a condition which not infrequently occurs in otherwise healthy people who have over-dosed themselves with an effervescent "hangover" remedy to shake off the effects, including alcoholic gastritis, of the night before.

6. Sleeping Pills

Such pills cloud the mind, slow reaction time, reduce awareness, and cause mental confusion; and when combined with alcohol can prove fatal. All sleeping pills are bad for pilots, and if you feel obliged to take them, then seek medical advice before you fly.

7. Sedatives and Tranquilisers

These, again, reduce awareness. Fear, which is an emotion

common to all human beings, is responsible for bringing a sense of danger to conscious level. These drugs can produce that slap-happy state of euphoric optimism which contains all the seeds of self-destruction.

8. Anti-Histamines

These drugs have found their way into many compound tablets used effectively in the treatment of such illnesses as hay fever, asthma, eczema and contact dermatitis. Anti-histamines, in combination with vaso-constricting drugs, are offered to the public as "Cold Cures". It should be realized that they are quite incapable of curing a cold, but are most effective in bringing about symptomatic relief whilst the body itself prepares to kill the virus which has caused the cold. Unfortunately, there is no anti-histamine which is free of side effects, and the one common to all is drowsiness. If you have reason to think that your particular brand of "Cold Cure" pill contains an anti-histamine, then consult your doctor before enjoying a lonely and perhaps permanent nap at 10000 ft.

9. Amphetamine Drugs

Drugs which are sold under such brand names as "Dexedrine", "Benzedrine", "Methedrine" and "Drinamyl" are used as appetite suppressants by the medical profession, and as pep pills by others. These drugs should be avoided, for over-dosage can cause over-confidence and give rise to headaches, giddiness and disorientation.

10. Antibiotic Drugs

Antibiotics are used to combat infection, and penicillin was the first of these powerful drugs to be discovered. In their short history of some twenty-five years this group of drugs has probably saved more lives than any other single group of medicines. They are unlikely to impair your flying ability—but those very conditions for which they are prescribed may be the cause of disabling symptoms.

11. Indigestion Remedies

Indigestion remedies which may contain **Anticholinergic Drugs** should be used with great caution and taken only under medical supervision, for many of these drugs contain sedatives and also have an atropine-like action which can affect the eyes and cause blurred vision. Pilots known to be suffering from a peptic ulcer are unfit for flying activities. A period of six weeks free of all symptoms should follow radiological evidence of healing before flying is again permitted.

12. Steroid Drugs

These are used in the treatment of many diseases which include such conditions as gout, asthma, hay fever and skin rashes. They are potent remedies—which can have serious side effects. These drugs should be taken only under strict medical supervision and flying activities should be discontinued until steroid therapy has ceased. Steroid ointments frequently prescribed for skin conditions can be used and are unlikely to produce adverse side effects.

13. The "Pill"

Currently being taken as a matter of routine by millions of women, the "pill" consists essentially of two female hormones. Some varieties are more likely than others to increase fluid retention and aggravate premenstrual tension. Emotional disturbances of this nature affect judgment and have been held responsible for accidents.

14. Motion Sickness Drugs

These can prove very successful in the prevention and treatment of vestibular-inspired nausea and vomiting. Their exact action is not understood and all have side reactions, and the one common to all is drowsiness. They should be used with great caution and taken only under medical supervision and must never be prescribed for the lone pilot.

Hyoscine Hydrobromide is offered to the public under the brand name of "Kwells". Each tablet contains 0·3 mg of the active ingredient, and is scored across the centre for easy division. Children tolerate this drug well and should be given between ¼ and ½ tablet according to age. It is, however, unsuitable for patients suffering from **Glaucoma.** The drug should be taken about 30 min before setting out on the journey. It is a relatively short-acting drug and its effects will wear off in about 4 to 6 hrs. Adults who are particularly sensitive to motion sickness may take two tablets at the start of the journey, and a further tablet every six hours. Hyoscine is the least likely of the motion sickness drugs to cause drowsiness. Although dryness of the mouth may be noticed with hyoscine, it remains probably the most effective and safest of the motion sickness drugs. The only disadvantage is its relatively short effective period of action.

Cyclizine Hydrochloride, 50 mg in tablet form, and supplied under the name of "Marzine", is also a most effective drug. Its action lasts for about 8 hr; however, it is more likely to cause drowsiness than hyoscine. It should not be taken by pregnant women during the first four months of pregnancy without first seeking medical advice.

Meclozine Hydrochloride, sold under the brand names of "Sea-Legs" in England and "Bonamine" in the United States, is also a potent anti-motion sickness drug, but should be taken with caution due to its sedative effect. Pregnant women should exercise the same caution as with "Marzine".

Promethazine Theoclate, 25 mg, is marketed under the trade name of "Avomine", whilst **Dimenhydrinate,** 50 mg, is available also in tablet form under the brand name of "Dramamine". Both are very satisfactory anti-motion sickness drugs, both are fairly long acting remedies, but both produce drowsiness in some subjects. Pregnant women should exercise the same precaution as with all the other tablets except "Kwells".

15. Innoculations and Vaccinations

These can cause delayed, and sometimes severe, side reactions and your doctor's advice should be sought before flying. While immunization against smallpox, yellow fever and cholera are recognized requirements for international travel, additional protection should be given against **Typhoid, Paratyphoid Fever, Tetanus** and **Poliomyelitis** to travellers intending to visit the tropics and certain continental countries.

The following scheme is suitable for pilots who are obliged to go abroad at short notice and wish to protect themselves against the more serious diseases by a course of prophylactic injections.

1st Day
1. Yellow Fever Injection.
2. Cholera Injection No. 1.
3. Oral Poliomyelitis No. 1.

5th Day
1. Smallpox Vaccination.
2. TABT Injection No. 1.

11th Day
Cholera Injection No. 2.

13th Day
Your Physician will want to read the result of your Smallpox Vaccination.

28th Day
1. TABT Injection No. 2.
2. Oral Poliomyelitis No. 2.

Oral Poliomyelitis No. 3 should be taken 4 weeks after Dose No. 2 and TABT Injection No. 3 should be given six to twelve months after Injection No. 2.

16. Dental Treatment

Where this has required the administration of a local or general anaesthetic, dental treatment will adversely affect ability to fly safely for at least twelve hours after they have been administered. An extraction performed to ease the pain of a dental abscess may, by causing a veritable avalanche of bacteria into the blood stream, give rise to a raised temperature and a feeling of general malaise, which could last several hours.

17. Drink

In small quantities alcohol relieves nervous tension and loosens the tongue, whilst in larger quantities it clouds the mind and causes mental confusion. Fly first and enjoy a drink later. In the context of Cupid, Shakespeare once said that alcohol provokes the desire but takes away the performance, and, medically speaking, it does precisely the same thing in the air, with equally disastrous results.

18. The Circadian Cycle

This rather intriguing title applies to an equally interesting mode of function of the human body. It is not by chance that man possesses a regular cycle of wakefulness and sleep. Each of us has an in-built endocrine clock which arouses us in the morning, prepares us for sleep at night and controls our metabolism during the day. Hormone production in the body rises and falls in a 24-hr cycle and the excretionary products of these various hormones may be found in the urine. Quantitative estimation of their presence may be related to bodily activity. When travelling, in an easterly or westerly direction, a jet aircraft may pass through several time zones in the course of a single flight. A watch may be instantly adjusted when passing through a time zone but not so the human body, which will require a period of twenty-four hours to adjust to a one hour time zone change. A person landing in New York after a flight from London will find that a period of five days will elapse before he can become fully adjusted psychologically and physiologically to the environment of his new time zone. It is interesting to note that the advent of the SST (Supersonic Transport) will solve many circadian problems over the north-Atlantic route. If the return journey is completed in one day it will be possible for crews and passengers alike to wake up and go to sleep in the same bed in the same place and in the same time zone after having passed through ten time zones change in the course of a round trip between London and New York.

19. Tranquility of Mind

Emphasis is rightly placed on the importance of physical fitness but it is equally true that the pilot's state of mind is probably one of the main factors responsible for unexplained accidents which are ultimately attributed to pilot error. A wise pilot avoids a row with his wife before he flies and delays giving any thought to his overdraft until he can discuss this with his Bank Manager after he has landed.

Most physical illnesses are clearly defined clinical entities, the nature of which is readily understood by the patient, who is usually most anxious to receive treatment and be restored to health. Unhappily, this state of affairs is often absent in the presence of mental illness, when the patient may even further complicate the issue by going to great lengths to hide his symptoms, in the foolish belief that to admit them would be to lose face in the eyes of his fellow men.

Otherwise healthy pilots may become mentally upset as a reaction to the everyday common stresses of life. These states of mind are usually transitory and disappear when the cause has been removed or when the patient has learned to come to terms with his problems. Symptoms associated with these states vary enormously and many manifest themselves in a physical form and give rise to such conditions as backache, fibrositis, flatulence, dyspepsia and diarrhoea. More commonly symptoms are of a purely mental nature, such as frontal headaches, agitation, depression, feelings of guilt and, most important of all and common to all these states, lack of concentration and loss of initiative. It is not unusual for symptoms to follow a patient's occupation and in the case of pilots may be expressed as vertigo, disorientation and a fear of flying.

The author had personal experience of such a case when flying in a service helicopter some years ago. The pilot suffered an attack of unexplained vertigo at 1200 ft in perfect visibility and was compelled to put the aircraft into auto-rotation and land on a beach near the Air Station. After a while he recovered his composure and flew the aircraft back to base, a distance of some two miles, and even during this short flight suffered another attack of vertigo. Subsequently, it transpired that this competent and experienced helicopter pilot, who was about to be released at the end of a short-service commission, had been suffering the wrath of a virago's tongue each time he returned home to his wife at the end of the day. It seemed that she felt that he was living on borrowed time and that he should give up flying and preserve his life in order to secure his release and accept his gratuity whilst still alive. Her constant nagging had broken him mentally, and the wretched fellow spent his last few weeks in the Royal Navy being interviewed by psychiatrists and doing a miserable desk job on the ground. The virago got her husband and his gratuity, but for how long she kept him I do not know.

Before flying and in the interests of flight safety a pilot should always coldly assess his current frame of mind and not regard himself as a man apart from other mortals. If worried or emotionally upset, do not fly alone and never act as Pilot-in-Command.

20. Don't Let Age Persuade You to Quit

When next you go down to the Social Security Office to draw your old-age pension ignore your wife's pleas to give up flying because you have become a senior citizen. Press on—an analysis of aircraft accidents involving older persons in the U.S.A. in 1965 reveals that this age group (over sixty) has an accident record essentially comparable, and in some cases superior, to that of the younger pilot! It is hardly credible, but in the year under review there was an old fellow still at it, a physician aged 93, and he had a valid Medical Certificate in his pocket to prove it.

wonderfull, I like it.

6. Survival

1. General Principles

When planning to fly over inhospitable regions of the earth you should seek expert advice, for this chapter has been written only as a guide to the basic principles of survival. Survival will be helped by—

(1) Rapid location
(2) Early rescue
(3) Maintenance of vitality and preservation of life until help arrives.

RAPID LOCATION

Provision of reliable equipment and observance of sensible precautions as summarized here will obviously help in simplifying and hence speeding up location—

(a) The installation of comprehensive radio, radio-navigational aids, and survival equipment aboard the aircraft.
(b) The precaution of filing a flight plan. However, do not omit to cancel this if the flight is postponed, and on landing at your destination do not forget to report your safe arrival to Air Traffic Control.
(c) Reporting your position at regular intervals throughout the flight to the appropriate Air Traffic Centre.
(d) Notifying immediately the appropriate Air Traffic Centre if for any reason the Flight Plan is changed whilst still airborne.

(*e*) In the event of making an emergency landing do all you can to establish contact with anyone, and give your position as clearly and as accurately as possible whilst you still have plenty of height in hand.

EARLY RESCUE

This will be largely dependent on one or both of the following—

(*a*) The availability of the Search and Rescue Services in the area.
(*b*) Your own ability to make easily visible ground signals or suitable radio signals, indicating your exact position to the rescue facility when it has reached your area.

MAINTENANCE OF VITALITY AND PRESERVATION OF LIFE UNTIL HELP ARRIVES

This depends upon many factors, and likely causes of death are—

(*a*) Lack of knowledge.
(*b*) Thirst.
(*c*) Starvation.
(*d*) Exposure.
(*e*) Heat exhaustion.
(*f*) Drowning.
(*g*) Injuries.
(*h*) Disease.

Provision of survival equipment is of first importance—but so also is a knowledge of its effective use, and the opportunities for improvization should also be borne in mind. Equipment may be considered as basic—for any journey—and additional—for particular journeys.

2. Survival Equipment Necessary for all Journeys

(*a*) Anti-glare spectacles to reduce the effect of sun, snow glare, sandstorms, etc.

(b) Hand mirror for signalling.

(c) Hand compass and maps.

(d) Locator beacon.

(e) Flares and dyes.

(f) Waterproof matches.

(g) Compact rations, including water.

(h) Additional clothing.

(j) A comprehensive **first-aid kit,** which must include drugs appropriate to the terrain; and light, easily inflatable splints to immobilize fractures of the fore-arm and leg.

(k) A whistle.

(l) A large knife of the Panga type.

3. Additional Equipment Necessary for Particular Journeys

DESERT TERRAIN

(a) Additional water.

(b) Collection of water from the desert itself. Dig a conical-shaped hole and place a tin can or some other suitable receiver at the bottom. Line the hole with an impermeable sheet as shown in Fig. 8. Polythene would serve as a very suitable material for this purpose.

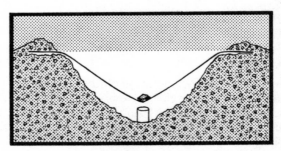

FIG. 8. Collection of Water from the Desert Itself

The edges of the polythene sheet are held down with sand and the apex of the cone should be lightly weighted to hold it above the can. Water from the sand is evaporated by the sun and condenses on the underside of the sheet and collects in the can.

(*c*) Solar still. This apparatus will produce an acceptable drinking fluid from brackish water and urine.

(*d*) Food should consist mostly of carbohydrates, such as glucose sweets and candies. Foods containing protein and fats increase fluid intake requirements.

(*e*) Always stay with your aircraft and use it to protect yourself from exposure at night and from heat exhaustion and loss of tissue fluids due to sweating during the day.

(*f*) Drinking water must be rationed on the following scale—

First day	None.
Subsequent Days	12–16 fl. oz. (350–500 ml) taken in equal amounts of 3–4 oz (90–120 ml) at 6-hr intervals. If this ration cannot be maintained, it should be reduced to 8 oz (250 ml) but no lower, with the exception that the last 8 oz (250 ml) can be split to last two days. When water is being taken, it should be sipped slowly, wetting the mouth before it is swallowed.

MOUNTAINOUS TERRAIN

(*a*) Additional clothing may be used to replace those garments which have become damp. Reference should be made to the protective measures against frostbite discussed on pp. 15 and 16.

(*b*) Build yourself a shelter. In very low temperatures an intact aircraft cabin may not offer sufficient protection and may even act like a refrigerator.

(*c*) Engine oil. Drain the sump as soon as possible, otherwise it may freeze, and add the oil to your equipment, for use as a smoke maker when signalling.

SHORT SEA CROSSINGS

Inflatable life jacket with integral locator beacon, dyes and flares.

LONG SEA CROSSINGS

(a) Inflatable life dinghy, in addition to a life jacket.

(b) The dinghy must contain an integral locator beacon, dyes, flares, de-salting tablets, water, dry clothing and fishing gear.

(c) An Immersion suit will provide protection from low sea temperatures, particularly during the period before the dinghy has been boarded, and together with the life jacket, will provide extra flotation. Once in the dinghy, the inflatable floor and apron with its hood should be deployed. Active measures must be taken to bale out any water from the dinghy and make it as dry as possible. Change into dry clothing, and weather permitting dry any clothes that have become wet.

(d) Sources of water may be—

1. Rain water.

2. Solar still.

3. Survival pack.

4. De-salting tablets, but do not forget that each tablet can only be used once.

5. If water has to be rationed, it should be allowed in slightly larger amounts than in the desert, but in the same sequence.

6. The body should be kept as cool as is compatible with comfort and health, in order to prevent loss of body fluids through sweating. Fish, if caught, should be taken in amounts of about 4 oz (120 g) daily, unless fresh water is freely available, because larger amounts, due to their salt content, increase the need for fluid intake.

7. Sea sickness can be a source of fluid loss and great distress, which may reduce the will to survive. Reference should be made to that section dealing with motion sickness on pp. 64 and 65.

JUNGLE TERRAIN

(a) *Malarial suppressant Drugs.* An acceptable drug for this purpose is Proguanil Hydrochloride, which is marketed under the brand name of "Paludrine". Two tablets (200 mg) should be taken daily, beginning one day prior to entering the malarial area and continuing throughout the period of exposure and for fourteen days after leaving the area.

(b) *Malarial Canopy Netting.* Always sleep under suitable netting if exposed to mosquitoes.

(c) Tropical Diarrheoa may be prevented or treated by taking Furazolidone, which is sold under the brand name of "Furoxone". Two tablets should be taken three times a day.

(d) Skin infections may be treated by the application of such compound ointments as Nystaform-H.C., which has anti-inflammatory, anti-bacterial and fungicidal properties, and is particularly satisfactory for the treatment of athlete's foot—a common condition in the jungle.

(e) More severe infections may be treated by various antibiotics, and oxytetracycline is an acceptable broad spectrum antibiotic for these purposes. It should be taken in the form of one tablet (250 mg) at 6-hr intervals.

(f) Anti-Snakebite packs should be carried.

(g) Insect Repellants.

(h) Water is likely to be plentiful but should be chlorinated by the addition of purifying tablets before being drunk. Clean water may be obtained from the severed ends of vines and bamboos.

(j) A length of 300 ft of nylon rope should be carried—for the height of jungle trees, if you land on them, may exceed 250 ft.

(*k*) In the event of a forced landing, do all you can to stall the aircraft on the tree tops, for in this position you will be more readily visible to search aircraft. If you crash through the heavy tree-top foliage, you will need a large Panga type knife to hack a clearing in the jungle, thus making yourself more visible from the air.

(*l*) Whenever possible stay with your aircraft. If you are forced to move away, remember to leave a clearly written note attached to your aircraft stating *when* you left and your *intended* compass heading, plus any other relevant information. Although you will probably not get very far, an attempt should be made to locate the nearest human community or reach the nearest river, whilst remembering most natives are friendly. Leave evidence of your passage through the jungle by marking the trees as you go. Inspect your exposed body surfaces at regular intervals for leeches. If these are present do not attempt to pull them off, but apply a lighted match or the burning end of a cigarette to their distal parts and they will fall off.

4. Escape by Parachute

Parachutes have been saving lives for a very long time. The first recorded case was that of a character called Jordaki Kuparenko, whose hot-air balloon burst into flames in the sky over Warsaw on a day in 1808. Like members of the Polish Air Force who flew so gallantly in the Second World War, Kuparenko was an intrepid fellow; he nipped over the side, opened his parachute and descended to safety before the astonished eyes of the worthy subjects of the Prince of Poland.

Private Pilots and many Glider Pilots are untrained in the use of parachutes. Under most circumstances, it is wise to deploy the canopy as soon as possible, when free of the aircraft, except perhaps when in a thunder cloud under circumstances mentioned in Chapter 4. The free-falling body will tend to spin, especially when in a back down attitude, and if this spinning movement is allowed to build up acceleration forces may cause disorientation and lead to fatal delay in operating the parachute assembly. The general rule, therefore, should take the spoken form— "Jump, One Thousand, Two Thousand, Pull Ripcord".

Having successfuly deployed his parachute the aviator should take up his landing attitude, at about 1000 ft, facing in the direction of drift. The legs and feet should be together, knees slightly bent, head well tucked in, and the arms, with the hands grasping the lift webs, should be at right-angles with the elbows held well forward. It is important not to pull the legs right up prior to impact with the ground, since this is likely to cause injuries to the pelvis and spine. It is best to look forward at an angle of about 45° and not straight down, since the latter view is liable to make the individual pull up his legs at the last moment. When the feet do touch the ground the body should be allowed to collapse in the direction in which the parachute is moving, thereby distributing the impact forces over a larger area of the body.

Those who successfully leap to safety by an Irving parachute are eligible for election to the Caterpillar Club. Medically speaking, this is an appropriate name in more senses than one, for caterpillars, insects, beetles and mammals up to the size of mice can leap out of aeroplanes and land quite unharmed without the aid of a parachute. It is all due to simple sums, for if one remembers that surface area has two dimensions and volume/weight has three it follows that surface area increases by the square and volume/weight by the cube. Thus, a creature weighs more in proportion to its surface area the bigger it becomes, and therefore the less will be its chances of surviving a fall from a flying machine. Whilst a mouse will be unharmed, a rat will be knocked out, a dog will be killed, a man will be broken, a horse will splash, and an elephant will disintegrate.

Happy Landings

Index